Nurses! Test Yourself in Pharmacology

Nurses! Test Yourself in ...

Nurses!
Test Yourself in
Pharmacology

Katherine M. A. Rogers

 Open University Press

Open University Press
McGraw-Hill Education
McGraw-Hill House
Shoppenhangers Road
Maidenhead
Berkshire
England
SL6 2QL

email: enquiries@openup.co.uk
world wide web: www.openup.co.uk

and Two Penn Plaza, New York, NY 10121–2289, USA

First published 2014

A catalogue record of this book is available from the British Library

ISBN-13: 978-0-33-524491-1
ISBN-10: 0-33-524491-2
eISBN: 978-0-33-524492-8

Library of Congress Cataloging-in-Publication Data
CIP data applied for

Typesetting and e-book compilations by
RefineCatch Limited, Bungay, Suffolk

Contents

ACKNOWLEDGEMENTS

I wish to thank Rachel Crookes and all the team at McGraw-Hill Education – Open University Press for all their help, support and patience throughout the writing of this book. I also wish to acknowledge the reviewers of the manuscript and in particular Dr. Noel Harris for his very useful feedback.

Finally, thank you to my husband Conor and son Rory for their endless patience and understanding.

ACKNOWLEDGEMENTS

ABOUT THE AUTHOR

Dr. Katherine Rogers is a lecturer in applied health sciences with the School of Nursing and Midwifery at Queen's University Belfast where she teaches health science subjects, including anatomy, physiology, pathophysiology and pharmacology to undergraduate and postgraduate nursing and midwifery students. She has written a number of peer-reviewed articles on health science education. She has held External Examiner posts in these subjects in a number of Higher Education Institutions across the UK. In 2011 she was awarded a Queen's University Belfast Rising Star Teaching Award for individual excellence in teaching.

Using this book

INTRODUCTION

Welcome to *Nurses! Test Yourself in Pharmacology*. I hope you find this an invaluable tool throughout your pharmacology course and beyond! The book is designed as a revision aid that you can use alongside your main textbook. Each chapter is designed for stand-alone revision, meaning that you need not read from the beginning to benefit from the book.

Each chapter begins with a brief introduction covering the main points of the topic and directing you to some useful resources. Some useful textbooks have been suggested that may support your recommended text; however, they should not replace the core reading for your course. The chapter then provides you with different types of questions that help you test your knowledge of the area. Do not ignore a question type if you are not tested in that way because the answer contains useful information that could easily be examined in an alternative question format. Answers are provided in each chapter with detailed explanations – this is to help you with revision but can also be used as a learning aid. A key feature of this book is the Drug Summary Diagrams at the end of some chapters, which present the key drugs discussed in the chapter according to their pharmacological classification. These diagrams have been designed to help you become familiar with the relationships between common drugs and how they may be used to treat a range of disorders often in more than one organ system.

A list of common abbreviations used throughout is provided at the front of the book, while a glossary of terms commonly used in pharmacology is provided at the back. All spellings and abbreviations used are in accordance with those published in the *British National Formulary* (BNF).

I hope that you enjoy using this book and that you find it a convenient and useful tool throughout your studies!

List of abbreviations

These are common abbreviations used in the clinical setting and throughout this book.

5-HT	serotonin	CVA	cerebrovascular accident (or stroke)
ABG	arterial blood gas		
ACE	angiotensin-converting enzyme	CVD	cardiovascular disease
		DKA	diabetic ketoacidosis
ACS	acute coronary syndrome	DM	diabetes mellitus
ADH	antidiuretic hormone (or vasopressin)	DMARD	disease-modifying antirheumatic drug
AIDS	acquired immune deficiency syndrome	DNA	deoxyribonucleic acid
		DPP-4	dipeptidylpeptidase-4
BAC	blood alcohol concentration	DVT	deep-vein thrombosis
		ECG	electrocardiogram
BNF	British National Formulary	EEG	electroencephalogram
		EMG	electromyography
BP	blood pressure	ESRF	(or ESRD) end-stage renal failure (or disease)
BSA	body surface area		
BUN	blood urea nitrogen	GABA	gamma-aminobutyric acid
CF	cystic fibrosis		
CHF	congestive heart failure	GFR	glomerular filtration rate
CK	creatinine kinase	GI	gastrointestinal
CO_2	carbon dioxide	GORD	gastro-oesophageal reflux disease
COCP	combined oral contraceptive pill		
		GP	general practitioner
COPD	chronic obstructive pulmonary disorder (or disease)	GTN	glyceryl trinitrate
		H_2	histamine$_2$
		HCl	hydrochloric acid
COX-1	cyclooxygenase-1	HDL	high-density lipoprotein
COX-2	cyclooxygenase-2	HIV	human immunodeficiency virus
CRF	chronic renal failure		
CSF	cerebrospinal fluid	HPV	human papilloma virus
CT	computerized tomography	HRT	hormone replacement therapy
CTS	carpal tunnel syndrome		

HSV	herpes simplex virus	PTH	parathyroid hormone
IBD	inflammatory bowel disorder (or disease)	RA	rheumatoid arthritis
		RAS	renin-angiotensin system
IBS	irritable bowel syndrome	RBC	red blood cell (erythrocyte)
ICP	intracranial pressure		
IV	intravenous	SERM	selective oestrogen receptor modulator
LDL	low-density lipoprotein		
		SNRI	serotonin and noradrenaline reuptake inhibiter
LP	lumbar puncture (or spinal tap)		
MAOI	monoamine-oxidase inhibitor	SSRI	selective serotonin reuptake inhibitor
MHRA	Medicines and Healthcare products Regulatory Agency	STEMI	ST-elevation myocardial infarction
		STI	sexually transmitted infection
MI	myocardial infarction (or heart attack)		
		t-PA	tissue plasminogen activator
MRI	magnetic resonance imaging	TBI	total body irradiation
MRSA	methicillin-resistant *Staphylococcus aureus*	TCA	tricyclic antidepressant
		TIA	transient ischaemic attack (or 'mini' stroke)
non-STEMI	non-ST-elevation myocardial infarction		
NSAID	non-steroidal anti-inflammatory drug	TKI	tyrosine kinase inhibitor
		TSH	thyroid-stimulating hormone
O_2	oxygen		
OTC	over-the-counter	UK	United Kingdom
PABA	para-aminobenzoic acid	USA	United States of America
PD	Parkinson's disease	UTI	urinary tract infection
PEFR	peak expiratory flow rate		
		UV	ultraviolet
PI	proteasome inhibitors	WBC	white blood cell (or leucocyte)
POM	prescription-only medicine		
		WHO	World Health Organization
PPI	proton pump inhibitor		

Common prefixes, suffixes and word roots

Prefix/suffix/ root	Definition	Example
a-/an	deficiency, lack of	*anuria = decrease or absence of urine production*
-aemia	of the blood	*ischaemia = decreased blood supply*
angio	vessel	*angiogenesis = growth of new vessels*
brady	slow	*bradycardia = slow heart beat*
broncho-	bronchus	*bronchitis = inflammation of the bronchus*
card-	heart	*cardiology = study of the heart*
chole-	bile or gallbladder	*cholecystitis = inflammation of the gallbladder*
cyto-	cell	*cytology = study of cells*
derm-	skin	*dermatology = study of the skin*
dys-	difficult	*dystocia = difficulty with delivery of fetal shoulders at birth*
-ema	swelling	*oedema = abnormal accumulation of tissue fluid*
entero-	intestine	*enteritis = inflammation of the intestinal tract*
erythro-	red	*erthyropenia = deficiency of red blood cells*
gast-	stomach	*gastritis = inflammation of stomach lining*
-globin	protein	*haemoglobin = iron-containing protein in the blood*
haem-/haemo-	blood	*haemocyte = a blood cell (especially red blood cell)*

hepat-	liver	*hepatitis = inflammation of the liver*
-hydr-	water	*rehydrate = replenish body fluids*
intra-	during	*intrapartum = during labour*
-itis	inflammation	*bronchitis = inflammation of the bronchus*
-kinesia	movement, motion	*bradykinesia = slow movements*
leuco-	white	*leucopenia = deficiency of white blood cells*
lymph-	lymph tissue/vessels	*lymphoedema = fluid retention in lymphatic system*
-lyso/-lysis	breaking down	*hydrolysis = breaking down molecule with water*
myo-	muscle	*myocardium = cardiac muscle*
nephro-	kidney	*nephritis = inflammation of the kidneys*
neuro-	nerve	*neurology = study of the nerves*
-ology	study of	*dermatology = study of the skin*
-oma	tumour	*lymphoma = tumour of the lymph tissue*
os-/osteo-	bone	*osteology = study of bones*
path-	disease	*pathology = study of disease*
-penia-	deficiency of	*leucopenia = deficiency of white blood cells*
pneumo-	air/lungs	*pneumonitis = inflammation of lung tissue*
tachy-	excessively fast	*tachycardia = excessive heart rate*
tox-	poison	*toxicology = study of poisons*
-uria	urine	*haematuria = blood in the urine*
vaso-	vessel	*vasoconstriction = narrowing of vessels*

Guide to textbook resources

Barber, P., Parkes, J. and Blundell, D. (2012) *Further Essentials of Pharmacology for Nurses*. Maidenhead: Open University Press.

Barber, P. and Robertson, D. (2012) *Essentials of Pharmacology for Nurses*, 2nd edition. Maidenhead: Open University Press.

Dale, M.M. and Haylett, D.G. (2009) *Pharmacology Condensed*, 2nd edition. Edinburgh: Churchill Livingstone.

Greenstein, B. and Gould, D. (2009) *Trounce's Clinical Pharmacology for Nurses*, 18th edition. Edinburgh: Churchill Livingstone.

Harris, N. and Shearer, D. (2012) *Nurses! Test Yourself in Non-Medical Prescribing*. Maidenhead: Open University Press.

Rogers, K.M.A. and Scott, W.N. (2011a) *Nurses! Test Yourself in Essential Calculation Skills*. Maidenhead: Open University Press.

Rogers, K.M.A. and Scott, W.N. (2011b) *Nurses! Test Yourself in Anatomy and Physiology*. Maidenhead: Open University Press.

Rogers, K.M.A. and Scott, W.N. (2011c) *Nurses! Test Yourself in Pathophysiology*. Maidenhead: Open University Press.

1 Introduction to pharmacology and drug administration

INTRODUCTION

Pharmacology is the study of drugs or chemicals used to treat and cure disease and their interactions in the body. Within the study of pharmacology there are a number of separate areas to consider, but for nurses the most important aspects are pharmacokinetics (PK) and pharmacodynamics (PD). Pharmacokinetics describes what the body does to a drug through the movement and distribution of that drug around the body. This is important because to be therapeutically useful, drugs must be absorbed into the body and transported to the desired site for action. Drugs will be therapeutically ineffective if they do not reach the target organ (site) to exert their activity. Pharmacodynamics considers what a drug does to the body – that is, the mechanism of drug action in the body. It describes the biochemical and physical effects of a drug and how it interacts with its desired target (such as a cell surface receptor, enzyme or DNA).

Nurses should understand the PK/PD principles of the drugs they are administering to patients. This includes the mode of action of drugs, dose responses, and potential interactions with other treatments (pharmacological or non-pharmacological) that the patient may be undergoing. Serious and adverse side-effects can arise from drug treatment (sometimes very quickly) and it is essential that the nurse can recognize these and act quickly to minimize their potential life-threatening effects.

Useful resources

Nurses! Test Yourself in Essential Calculation Skills
Chapters 1 and 2

Nurses! Test Yourself in Anatomy and Physiology
Chapters 1 and 2

Nurses! Test Yourself in Non-Medical Prescribing
Chapters 4 and 6

LABELLING EXERCISE

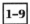 Identify the routes of administration in Figures 1.1 and 1.2 using the terms provided in the box below

intramuscular	rectal	intradermal
oral	subcutaneous	intravenous
topical	inhalation	transdermal

Figure 1.1 Common routes for the administration of medicines

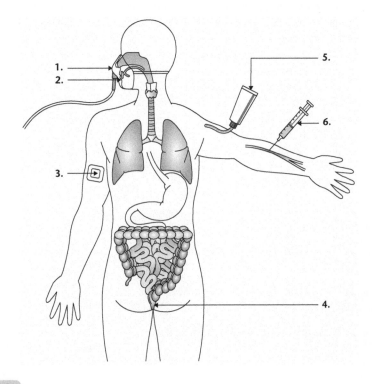

Figure 1.2 Position of the needle for common injection routes

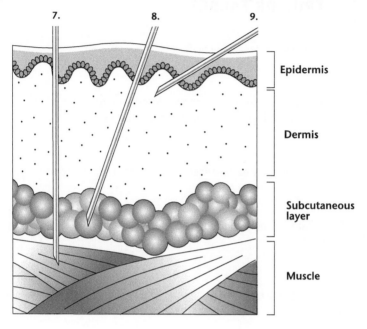

TRUE OR FALSE?

Are the following statements true or false?

10 In pharmacology, the word 'agonist' describes a drug that binds or inter-acts with its biological receptor but produces no effect.

11 An antagonist may be described as competitive or non-competitive.

12 The pharmacological action of a drug varies significantly among individuals.

13 A pro-drug describes a drug that is pharmacologically inactive until it reaches the liver and is metabolized.

14 Drugs administered intravenously (IV) are considered to have 100% absorption into the systemic circulation.

15 Free, unbound drug molecules cannot exert a pharmacological effect.

16 Most drugs are excreted in the urine.

MULTIPLE CHOICE

Identify one correct answer for each of the following.

17 The time required for the onset of a drug's action depends on its delivery to the site of action. Which of the following is not an important consideration in drug delivery?

a) route of administration

b) rate of absorption

c) rate of elimination

d) distribution of drug

18 How many factors are associated with a drug's distribution?

a) 1

b) 2

c) 3

d) 4

19 Which of the following describes the amount of drug absorbed by the body and distributed systemically?

a) bioavailability

b) first-pass metabolism

c) biotransformation

d) pharmacokinetics

20 Most drugs and drug molecules are excreted by the:

a) liver

b) kidneys

c) gall bladder

d) lungs

21 The ability of the kidneys to excrete drugs is called:

a) renal excretion

b) renal filtration

c) renal secretion

d) renal clearance

22 The time taken for the concentration of a drug to fall to half its original level is called:

a) half-life

b) steady state

c) elimination

d) clearance

23 When the amount of drug excreted equals the amount being absorbed, the condition is called:

a) toxicity

b) half-life

c) therapeutic limit

d) steady state

24 Sometimes drug metabolism processes become more effective, which can lead to:

a) drug toxicity

b) drug tolerance

c) drug overdose

d) liver failure

FILL IN THE BLANKS

Fill in the blanks in each statement using the options in the box below.
Not all of them are required, so choose carefully!

urine	faeces
receptors	formulation
enzymes	concentration
slowly	lipid solubility
enterohepatic recirculation	carriers
perfusion	specificity
infusion	first-pass metabolism
ion channels	distribution
water solubility	affinity
second-pass metabolism	systemic circulation

25 Drug _____ describes how well a drug binds to its specific target.

26 The ability of drugs to cross cell membranes depends on their _____
_____ .

27 Tissue _____ has a significant role in the initial distribution of a
drug.

28 The physical and chemical composition of a drug is called its
_____ .

29 Drugs direct their effects at molecular targets within the body. The four most common molecular targets are: _____, _____, and _____ _____.

30 The products of bilary excretion are eliminated from the body via the _____.

31 Some drugs undergo _____ _____, which prolongs their effect.

32 _____ – _____ _____ occurs in the liver.

33 Sustained release drugs are delivered _____ into the blood.

ANSWERS

 LABELLING EXERCISE

Figure 1.3 Common routes for the administration of medicines

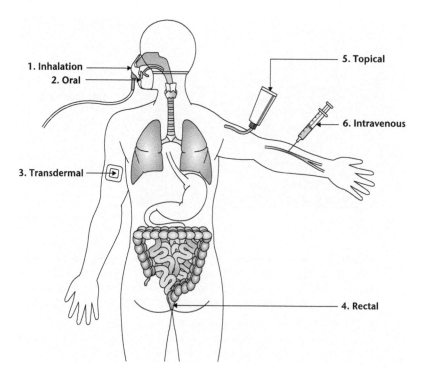

1. Inhalation
2. Oral
3. Transdermal
4. Rectal
5. Topical
6. Intravenous

Figure 1.4 Position of the needle for common injection routes

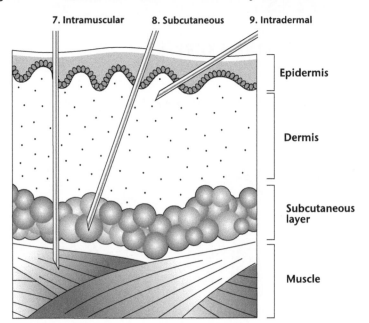

1   **Inhalation:** drugs targeting the respiratory tract may be inhaled to produce a rapid, local effect on the respiratory system. Drugs that are absorbed by the lungs to produce a general effect may also be administered by inhalation (for example, some general anaesthetics).

2   **Oral:** this is the most common route of administration because it is the easiest for both the patient and the person administering the medicine. There are many formulations available for the oral administration of drugs, including tablets, capsules, caplets, elixirs, linctus, lozenges, oral powders, and suspensions. The absorption of orally administered medicines is affected by several factors, including:

- the drug formulation
- the presence of food in the stomach
- the rate of gastric emptying
- possible drug interactions (especially if drugs are administered together).

The formulation of tablets, capsules, and caplets affects the absorption of drugs; for example, many enteric-coated tablets are now available to protect the lining of the stomach by preventing the release of the active ingredient until it reaches the duodenum. Sublingual tablets are placed under the tongue for absorption, while buccal tablets are administered between the cheek and gum. Like tablets, capsules and caplets deliver a measured dose of medication (for example 250 mg), although capsules and caplets are generally considered easier to swallow than tablets. They differ in their shape and rate of absorption of the medicine each contains. A capsule has a cylindrical-shaped shell (often made of gelatine), while a caplet is an oval (or capsule)-shaped tablet. Elixirs are alcohol-based solutions. A lozenge is designed to dissolve slowly in the mouth, since it is absorbed here it generally has a local effect. A linctus is a sweet, sucrose syrup often prescribed when administering drugs to children who may find it difficult to swallow tablets; a sugar-free formulation is preferable when available. An oral powder is usually dissolved in juice or water before administration, while an oral suspension is mixed with, but not completely dissolved in, a liquid. It must be shaken before administration to distribute and suspend the drug particles equally. A disadvantage of liquid preparations over solid dosage forms is that liquid preparations rely on the patient, carer or other administrator to measure the dose accurately and subsequently could result in the incorrect dose being given.

3 *Transdermal:* active drug ingredients may be delivered via the skin for systemic distribution, often using a transdermal patch. For example, nicotine patches are used in nicotine replacement therapy as a smoking cessation aid. A transdermal analgesic patch (such as buprenorphine or fentanyl) may be applied to the skin to relieve moderate to severe pain.

4 *Rectal:* certain drugs may be absorbed from the rectum and may be administered as a suppository or enema. A suppository is a bullet-shaped formulation that melts at body temperature, dispersing the drug. The drug in an enema is suspended in a solution and infused into the rectum. This route is useful to avoid first-pass metabolism (see Answer 19).

5 *Topical (local):* drugs may be applied topically (locally) to the skin, mucous membranes or surface wounds, usually in the form of creams, ointments or gels. Topically applied medicines are primarily active at the site of application, although some drugs (for example, non-steroidal anti-inflammatory drugs (NSAIDs)) are also absorbed into the systemic circulation and can therefore cause side-effects.

6 *Intravenous (IV):* this route has the most rapid action since the drug is applied directly into the bloodstream and has a bioavailability of 100% (see Answers 14 and 19). It may be used for drugs that are too irritating to be administered intramuscularly. This procedure is technically quite difficult and the nurse must be careful not to inadvertently inject into an artery, which can lead to arterial spasm and tissue damage.

7 *Intramuscular (IM):* this route is easier than the intravenous one but can be quite painful, so the maximum volume for delivery depends on the muscle being injected. Some common muscles should only receive 1mL intramuscular injection. Higher volumes may be injected depending on muscle size and its capacity to cope with the volume being injected. Absorption from the site is variable and depends on the blood flow but can be increased by exercise and rubbing the injection site. Usually absorption is greatest from the deltoid muscle and least from the buttock.

8 **Subcutaneous (SC):** this route is widely used. The common areas for subcutaneous injections are the forearm, outer aspect of the thigh or the abdominal wall. Absorption is slower than with an intramuscular injection (see Figure 1.5) and the area should not be massaged after administration. When a local effect is required (for example, with a local anaesthetic), a vasoconstrictor may be added to the injection to narrow the blood vessels and prevent the drug being distributed away from the site of injection.

Figure 1.5 The effect of route of administration on plasma concentrations of drug after one dose

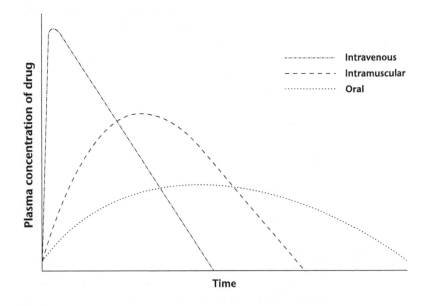

9 **Intradermal (ID):** this is the route often used when administering immunizations. A very small volume is injected at an angle, just under the skin in the dermis, commonly in the upper arm. The injection site should not be massaged when the needle is removed.

TRUE OR FALSE?

10 **In pharmacology, the word 'agonist' describes a drug that binds or interacts with its biological receptor but produces no effect.**

An agonist is a drug that binds to, or interacts with, its specific biological receptor (such as a cell surface receptor, an enzyme or a section of DNA), stimulating the receptor to trigger a response by the cell. The response is produced in a similar manner to that of the natural physiological ligand (or chemical), such as a hormone or neurotransmitter – that is, the action of an agonist mimics that of the receptor's natural ligand (see Figure 1.6). For example, a beta$_2$ (β_2) agonist drug (such as salbutamol) mimics the action of the natural ligand for the β_2 adrenergic receptors (for example adrenaline) on the muscles surrounding the airways. Activation of β_2 adrenergic receptors relaxes the muscles surrounding the airways, causing bronchodilation, which opens the airways. Dilation of the airways helps to relieve the symptoms of dyspnoea (shortness of breath).

Figure 1.6 Mechanism of ligand/agonist–receptor binding

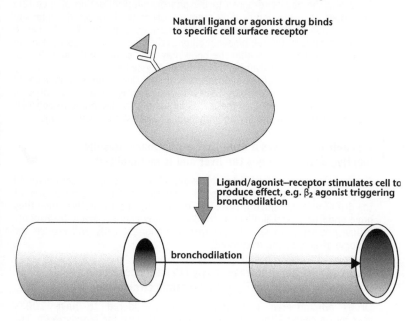

Natural ligand or agonist drug binds to specific cell surface receptor

Ligand/agonist–receptor stimulates cell to produce effect, e.g. β_2 agonist triggering bronchodilation

bronchodilation

11   **An antagonist may be described as competitive or non-competitive.**

An antagonist drug may compete with the natural ligand to bind with the cell surface receptor. When it binds with the natural ligand an antagonist will not produce a cellular response, thus an antagonist inhibits the action of the natural ligand. Sometimes the inhibition of the cellular response is desirable in therapeutics and many drugs utilize this mode of action. For example, the cells of some breast cancer patients possess many receptors that will bind to the natural oestrogen hormone circulating in the body. Since oestrogen stimulates breast cancer cells to grow, the continued binding of oestrogen to these receptors will allow the cancerous cells to multiply rapidly, enabling the malignant tumour to grow and spread. Competitive antagonists work by competing with the natural oestrogen ligand to bind with the receptor and once bound they inhibit the cellular response. When the competitive antagonist drug is bound to the receptor, it effectively blocks the oestrogen receptors on the cell surface, which prevents the natural oestrogen ligands from binding to the same receptors and hence tumour cell growth is prohibited. This is how a 'competitive antagonist' works. Tamoxifen is an example of a competitive antagonist used in the treatment of breast cancer.

12   **The pharmacological action of a drug varies significantly among individuals.**

Generally, the body's response to the pharmacological action of a certain drug does not vary significantly among individuals; however, the intensity and duration of the drug response may vary considerably. This is due to two main factors: (1) the bioavailability of the drug (plasma concentration of the absorbed drug) within the body may vary significantly, and (2) the sensitivity and responsiveness of the necessary cell surface receptors may differ. Usually these individual differences are not significant enough to cause concern, although some drugs have a narrow margin between therapeutic effect and toxicity and with these it is important for the nurse to consider the factors that may modify an individual's response to specific drugs.

13   **A pro-drug describes a drug that is pharmacologically inactive until it reaches the liver and is metabolized.**

A pro-drug may be used if the bioavailability of the orally administered drug is quite poor. It may also be used to increase the selectivity of the drug for its intended target. Pro-drugs only become active when they have undergone metabolism in the liver. Many chemotherapy treatments utilize pro-drugs to specifically target malignant cells and reduce the adverse effects of the treatment.

14   **Drugs administered intravenously (IV) are considered to have 100% absorption into the systemic circulation.**

Drugs administered intravenously are considered to have 100% absorption because they are delivered directly into the bloodstream. The blood plasma concentration of orally administered drugs is compared

against the concentration of the same I V-administered drug to determine
the bioavailability of the oral dosage.

15 **Free, unbound drug molecules cannot exert a
pharmacological effect.**

Drugs are considered free and unbound when they are not bound to
plasma proteins in the blood. Only free drug molecules, which are not
bound to plasma proteins, can leave the bloodstream and enter the
interstitial (tissue) fluid to exert a pharmacological effect. While bound
to plasma proteins such as albumin, drug molecules cannot leave the
blood and therefore remain pharmacologically unreactive (inert).

16 **Most drugs are excreted in the urine.**

Most drugs are excreted in the urine either unchanged or as a metabolite.
Three renal processes are involved in excretion of drugs. In the first
stage, glomerular filtration, small drug molecules are forced across the
membrane of the glomerulus by the high pressure in the renal arteries
and enter the filtrate in the renal tubule at a concentration equal to that
of the blood plasma. Drugs bound to plasma proteins are not filtered. As
water is reabsorbed from the filtrate, the concentration of drug in the
urine increases. Drug molecules that are not filtered out of the blood in
the glomerulus are secreted into the filtrate in the proximal convoluted
tubule. The process of secretion is highly effective and can remove most
of the drug from the blood in just one passage through the kidneys. Other
routes of excretion include the lungs and biliary excretion.

a b c d MULTIPLE CHOICE

Correct answers identified in bold italics.

17 **The time required for the onset of a drug's action depends on
its delivery to the site of action. Which of the following is not an
important consideration in drug delivery?**

a) route of administration   b) rate of absorption
c) *rate of elimination*   d) distribution of drug

For many drugs, the time taken for the onset of drug action is an
important consideration because its desired effect is required within a
certain timeframe. The time to the onset of drug action can be modified
in a number of ways. For example, if drug action is required quickly
an intramuscular or intravenous route of administration may be taken.
For patients who suffer chronic pain, analgesia (pain relief) may be
administered through a transdermal patch which provides a more
continuous plasma drug level to control the pain and reduce the amount
of oral medication required; this is particularly important in older adults
and patients who may have difficulty swallowing tablets or capsules. The

rate of drug elimination will determine the duration of the drug effect: the quicker the drug is removed from its target site, the shorter the drug's therapeutic effect.

18 How many factors are associated with a drug's distribution?

a) 1   b) 2   c) 3   **d) 4**

Once a drug has been administered and absorbed by the body, it must be distributed to the correct site of action. For some drugs the desired site of action is known (thus a drug may be administered locally at the site) but when the site of action is unknown, drugs must be distributed systemically (throughout the body) to ensure they reach the necessary target. Four factors need to be considered regarding drug distribution in the body: (1) distribution into the body fluids; (2) uptake of drugs by body tissues (organs); (3) the extent of plasma protein binding; and (4) passage through barriers (such as the blood–brain barrier).

19 Which of the following describes the amount of drug absorbed by the body and distributed systemically?

a) bioavailability   b) first-pass metabolism

c) biotransformation   d) pharmacokinetics

Bioavailability refers to the quantity of the administered drug that is absorbed into the body and distributed by the systemic blood circulation. Bioavailability is affected by incomplete absorption and first-pass metabolism, so the route of administration is significant in determining the bioavailability of a drug. For example, drugs that are administered orally may not be fully absorbed from the stomach or intestinal tract (if there is a lot of food present or there is GI disturbance), which will reduce the amount of drug entering the bloodstream. Some drugs are significantly metabolized in their first transit through the liver (first-pass metabolism), which also reduces bioavailability (see Answer 32). Drugs administered intravenously are considered to have 100% absorption (because they are delivered directly into the bloodstream) and so the blood plasma concentration of orally administered drugs is compared against the concentration of IV-administered drugs to determine the bioavailability of the oral dosage. Biotransformation describes the metabolism of drugs in the body. It mainly occurs in the liver. Pharmacokinetics describes what the body does to drugs from administration to excretion.

20 Most drugs and drug molecules are excreted by the:

a) liver   **b) kidneys**   c) gall bladder   d) lungs

Excretion of drugs occurs primarily through the kidneys, although small quantities of drug may be detected in the faeces. Drugs that are detected in the faeces are eliminated from the body through the bile. Drugs may also be detected in sweat, saliva, hair, tears, and exhaled air, although these are not considered routes of excretion since the quantities usually detectable are very low.

21 | The ability of the kidneys to excrete drugs is called:

a) renal excretion   b) renal filtration
c) renal secretion   **d) *renal clearance***

Renal clearance is determined by dividing the amount of drug excreted in the urine by the plasma concentration of the drug. In a healthy adult, the kidneys filter 120 mL of plasma every minute. Based on this figure, if a drug has a renal clearance value considerably lower than 120 mL per minute, it means the drug is either (1) not well filtered as it passes through the glomeruli of the kidneys or (2) the drug is filtered and then mostly reabsorbed into the plasma at the kidney tubules. Renal clearance values of more than 120 mL per minute indicate that the drug is filtered by the glomeruli and actively secreted by the tubules. Drugs with high renal clearance values rely on the healthy functioning kidneys to eliminate them from the body, otherwise the drug will accumulate in the body – this is particularly important when prescribing such drugs to patients with kidney disease or individuals at risk of renal complications from other illnesses (such as diabetes). Drugs with low renal clearance rates rely on other elimination mechanisms, usually by the liver in the bile. Doses of drugs with low renal clearance need not be modified for patients with kidney disease. The renal clearance rate in newborn babies and older adults is significantly lower and these patients need to receive lower drug doses (see Chapter 12).

22 | The time taken for the concentration of a drug to fall to half its original level is called:

a) *half-life* b) steady state c) elimination d) clearance

The half-life (or elimination half-life) of a drug is the time taken for the plasma concentration of a drug to decrease by half. The half-life indicates the speed of elimination of a drug and therefore implies the duration of action of a drug. The faster the elimination of a drug, the shorter its half-life will be because plasma concentrations will decrease relatively quickly (see Figure 1.7). When the half-life of a drug is known, it can be used to help determine the intervals between drug doses in patients.

23 | When the amount of drug excreted equals the amount being absorbed, the condition is called:

a) toxicity b) half-life c) therapeutic limit **d) *steady state***

Ideally a therapeutic effective concentration of a drug (or steady state) would be achieved and maintained with a single dose. Unfortunately this is rarely possible so to maintain a steady state, doses have to be administered at intervals. A steady state may be reached quickly by initially administering a higher dose of the drug – known as a loading dose – followed by a maintenance dose. Some antibiotics are administered using this loading–maintenance dose regimen to rapidly attack bacteria and produce desired levels of the drug in the body immediately to combat infection. Rapidly excreted drugs (with relatively short half-lives) require frequent administration or a continuous infusion to maintain a reasonably steady state in the body (see Figure 1.8).

Figure 1.7 The half-life of a drug after one IV injection

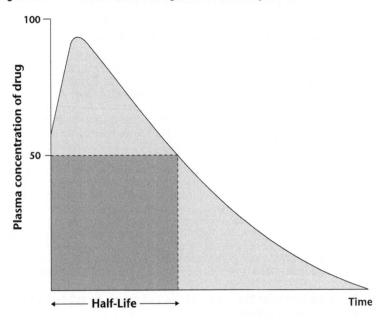

Figure 1.8 Influence of excretion on achieving a steady-state blood concentration of a drug

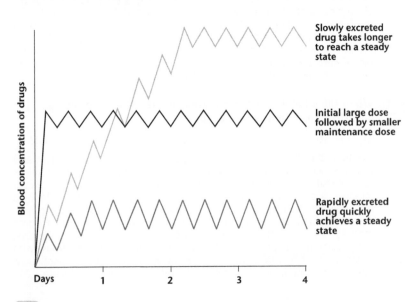

24 **Sometimes drug metabolism processes become more effective, which can lead to:**

a) drug toxicity

b) *drug tolerance*

c) drug overdose

d) liver failure

Drug tolerance may develop when the metabolic processes become more effective. In this situation, repeatedly larger doses of the drug will be required to produce the same therapeutic effect. Patients taking anti-epileptic drugs can sometimes develop drug tolerance, so their initial prescriptions should be as low a dose as necessary to control seizures and still allow for an increased dose in the future.

FILL IN THE BLANKS

25 **Drug *affinity* describes how well a drug binds to its specific target.**

Drugs with a high affinity bind preferentially to their specific physiological target compared with other drug molecules that may be present. The higher the affinity, the tighter the drug will bind to its target. Even low concentrations of very high affinity drugs will bind to their targets preferentially, which can be useful with drugs that are toxic at higher doses.

26 **The ability of drugs to cross cell membranes depends on their *lipid solubility*.**

Lipid-soluble drugs can easily enter cells from the interstitial (tissue) fluid by crossing the cell membranes. This is due to the phospholipid nature of cell membranes, which separates the intracellular and extracellular fluid compartments and facilitates the movement of lipids through the cell membrane. Water-soluble drugs will not cross cell membranes as easily. Due to their relatively favourable solubility, lipid-soluble drugs (such as warfarin) will be widely distributed throughout the body fluids and compartments, whereas the distribution of water-soluble drugs tends to be restricted to the extracellular fluid compartments of the plasma and interstitial fluid.

27 **Tissue *perfusion* has a significant role in the initial distribution of a drug.**

Organs and tissues that are richly perfused with blood will initially receive more drug molecules than regions that do not have a rich blood supply. This is because the drug molecules are transported around the body in the blood, so that areas such as the brain, heart, and kidneys, which receive a rich supply of blood, will initially receive more drug molecules quickly. Bone and adipose (fat) tissue are less well perfused and therefore receive less drug during the initial distribution; even very lipid-soluble drugs will not initially be detected in significant quantities in adipose tissue. After initial distribution, drugs become redistributed to the tissues for which they have highest affinity.

28 **The physical and chemical composition of a drug is called its** *formulation*.

The formulation of a drug describes all physical and chemical aspects of a medicine, including the active ingredients and any excipients (inactive substances that serve as the vehicle or medium for a drug). Excipients can be responsible for adverse drug reactions and may vary between brands, therefore the rate of release of the active ingredient may be different.

29 **Drugs direct their effects at molecular targets within the body. The four most common molecular targets are:** *receptors*, *enzymes*, *carriers*, **and** *ion channels*.

Many drugs target and bind to protein molecules located on cell membranes. The phospholipid bilayer of the cell membrane is selectively permeable and has protein molecule receptors embedded throughout the surface that facilitate the movement of substances in and out of the cell. Certain molecules called ligands bind to specific receptors and produce a response. Drugs may bind to receptors agonistically to mimic the response of a natural ligand or antagonistically to inhibit the natural response. Salbutamol and morphine are examples of common drugs that interact with receptors. Many drugs act by targeting natural enzymes and inhibiting their activity. For example, angiotensin converting enzyme (ACE) inhibitor drugs reduce blood pressure by preventing the action of angiotensin converting enzyme which converts angiotensin I to angiotensin II. In the absence of angiotensin II, blood pressure falls. Carrier proteins (or transport systems) may be targeted by drugs to prevent the normal physiological recycling of certain chemical transmitters. An example is the inhibition of the re-uptake of the neurotransmitter serotonin by certain antidepressant drugs, causing an accumulation of serotonin at the synapse, which enhances mood. Ion channels in the cell membrane may be targeted by drugs in two ways: (1) channels are blocked, as in calcium channel blockers, which block the entry of calcium into cells, or (2) channels may be regulated by drugs that bind to the channel, altering the channel's response to its normal target.

30 **The products of bilary excretion are eliminated from the body via the** *faeces*.

Drugs are often broken down or combined with other chemicals by enzymes in the liver making them inactive. These metabolites then pass out of the liver, mix with the bile, and enter the gastrointestinal (GI) tract. They pass through the GI tract with other unwanted products and are eventually eliminated from the body in the faeces.

31 Some drugs undergo <u>enterohepatic</u> <u>recirculation</u>, which prolongs their effect.

During bilary excretion, some drugs are reabsorbed from the GI tract back into the blood and travel to the liver again where they are further metabolized. This helps to maintain constant circulating levels of the drug, which prolongs the drug's effect until the next dose is administered. The combined oral contraceptive pill (COCP) is an example of a drug that undergoes this process; this enables the COCP to maintain constant high levels of the hormones required to prevent fertilization of the egg or implantation of a fertilized egg, thus preventing pregnancy. It is also the reason why the COCP should be taken at the same time each day.

32 <u>First-pass</u> <u>metabolism</u> occurs in the liver.

The first-pass metabolism (or effect) describes the breakdown (metabolism) of drugs by enzymes in the liver before the drug has entered the general circulation. After an oral drug is absorbed in the digestive tract, it passes to the liver via the hepatic portal vein. A family of enzymes in the liver, known as cytochrome P450 (or microsomal) enzymes, specialize in metabolism and certain enzymes within the family target drugs for metabolism. Each time a drug passes through the liver, it undergoes a certain amount of metabolism, which varies depending on the drug. The amount of metabolism the drug undergoes during its first passage through the liver will determine how much of the drug actually enters the circulation (known as the drug's bioavailability). If a drug undergoes extensive first-pass metabolism in the liver, very little of the drug will remain when it is released into the circulation, which will limit its therapeutic efficacy. The anti-angina medicine, glyceryl trinitrate (GTN), is a drug that undergoes almost complete first-pass metabolism, which is why it is usually administered sublingually. From this site, it is directly absorbed into the blood, which gives it sufficient time to exert its therapeutic effect before it is metabolized in the liver. Each time a drug passes through the liver, it undergoes further metabolism by the cytochrome P450 enzymes. Some drugs induce certain cytochrome P450 enzymes, which increases their metabolic activity; while other drugs inhibit specific cytochrome P450 enzymes, which reduces their metabolic activity. This is the basis for many drug interactions (see Chapter 13).

33 Sustained release drugs are delivered <u>slowly</u> into the blood.

Sustained (prolonged) release formulations are delivered slowly, but at a steady rate, into the blood. This maintains a prolonged therapeutic action. It usually means a patient requires fewer tablets (if the drug is in tablet form) and side-effects may be reduced because peak plasma levels of the drug are reduced.

2 Drugs associated with infection, inflammation, and pain

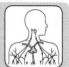

INTRODUCTION

The body has developed very efficient mechanisms to protect itself from infection by invading pathogens. The inflammatory response is part of the innate immune system's non-specific reaction to injury or infection. When the body is not able to overcome invading pathogens, an infection may arise which can be local to a certain area or it may spread systemically throughout the body.

A wide range of drugs target the cells and chemicals of the inflammatory response to reduce inflammation and the associated pain that accompanies inflammation, including the non-steroidal anti-inflammatory drugs (NSAIDs) and corticosteroid agents. Other types of pain medication, such as paracetamol and the opioid-type therapies, exploit the body's natural analgesic pathway to prevent the body from interpreting pain signals but do not reduce inflammation.

Nurses must consider the degree of pain and inflammation a patient is experiencing to ensure the appropriate type of medication is being administered. It is also important to consider the best route of administration based on the location of pain or inflammation and the dose of medication necessary for a therapeutic effect. The nurse should be aware of any other conditions the patient may have, or medications that the patient may be taking, to be confident that pain or anti-inflammatory medications being administered are appropriate and safe.

Useful resources

Nurses! Test Yourself in Pathophysiology
Chapters 1 and 2

Nurses! Test Yourself in Essential Calculation Skills
All chapters

Essentials of Pharmacology for Nurses, 2nd edition
Chapter 5

TRUE OR FALSE?

Are the following statements true or false?

1 The main target of NSAIDs is the cyclooxygenase-1 enzyme.

2 Anti-inflammatory corticosteroids inhibit the action of the natural glucocorticosteroids.

3 Compound analgesics contain simple analgesia and a low-dose opioid.

4 Patients on long-term corticosteroid treatment are at risk of serious side-effects.

5 Antibacterial drugs target bacterial cells in the human body but do not harm human cells.

6 The threadworm is a relatively common cause of helminth infection in the UK, especially in children.

7 Gram-positive bacteria will not absorb the purple-coloured Gram stain.

8 Broad-spectrum antibacterials should only be prescribed when the type of bacterial causing an infection is known.

MULTIPLE CHOICE

Identify one correct answer for each of the following.

9 The recommended adult dose of oral paracetamol is:

a) 0.25–0.5 g, no more than 2 g in 24 hours

b) 0.5–1.0 g, no more than 2 g in 24 hours

c) 0.25–0.5 g, no more than 4 g in 24 hours

d) 0.5–1.0 g, no more than 4 g in 24 hours

10 Paracetamol may be described as:

a) anti-inflammatory and non-steroidal

b) non-anti-inflammatory and non-steroidal

c) anti-inflammatory and steroidal

d) non-anti-inflammatory and steroidal

11 A major structural difference between bacterial and human cells is:

a) bacterial cells have a cell wall

b) bacterial cells have no nucleus

c) bacterial cells have multiple nuclei

d) there are no differences

12 Which of the following types of antibacterials is not a part of the beta-lactam family?

a) penicillins

b) carbapenems

c) cephalosporins

d) tetracyclines

13 The most serious side-effect associated with penicillins is:

a) nausea and vomiting

b) diarrhoea

c) anaphylaxis

d) drowsiness

14 Which of the following antibacterials may be used in patients who are penicillin-hypersensitive?

a) erythromycin

b) amoxicillin

c) benzylpenicillin

d) co-amoxiclav

15 Which of the following ribosome-targeting antibacterials is not well absorbed when administered orally?

a) tetracyclines

b) aminoglycosides

c) chloramphenicol

d) erythromycin

16 This group of antibacterial agents interferes with folic acid synthesis by bacteria:

a) fluoroquinolones

b) beta-lactams

c) tetracyclines

d) sulphonamides

17 Which of the following type of drugs is not considered part of the 'analgesic ladder'?

a) strong opioids

b) mild opioids

c) $beta_2$ agonists

d) non-opioids

FILL IN THE BLANKS

Fill in the blanks in each statement using the options in the box below.
Not all of them are required, so choose carefully!

chronic inflammatory	coronary heart
protozoal	antimicrobial
antibiotic	sympathomimetics
viral	beta-lactamase
fluoroquinolone	corticosteroids
opioids	tetracyclines
penicillins	

18 _____ are anti-inflammatory drugs that reduce inflammation and suppress immune responses.

19 Selective cyclooxygenase-2 inhibitors may be used to treat _____ _____ diseases.

20 Antibacterials, antifungals, antiprotozoals, and antivirals all belong to the _____ family of drugs.

21 Toxoplasmosis and trichomoniasis are the most common _____ infections in the U K.

22 _____ _____ is an enzyme produced by resistant bacteria that makes antibacterial drugs ineffective.

23 _____ bind to a number of ions and metals, which inhibits their absorption.

24 The _____ family of antibacterials inhibits DNA replication and protein synthesis.

25 _____ produce analgesia by acting on the central nervous system.

ANSWERS

TRUE OR FALSE?

1 **The main target of NSAIDs is the cyclooxygenase-1 enzyme.**

The primary target of NSAIDs is the cyclooxygenase-2 (COX-2) enzyme, which is only produced during the inflammatory response and therefore mainly found in inflamed tissue. COX-2 stimulates the production of the main inflammatory prostaglandin (prostaglandin E_2). Therefore, suppressing the production of this prostaglandin by inhibiting COX-2 activity will help reduce inflammation and the associated pain. The COX-1 enzyme is responsible for producing non-inflammatory prostaglandins, which are found throughout the body and are involved in maintaining tissue homeostasis. COX-1 and COX-2 are structurally very similar, so a number of NSAIDs will inhibit the action of both enzymes rather than just COX-2 in inflamed tissues. This inhibition of the non-inflammatory COX-1 is why certain side-effects such as gastrointenstinal disturbances are associated with some NSAIDs.

2 **Anti-inflammatory corticosteroids inhibit the action of the natural glucocorticosteroids.**

Anti-inflammatory corticosteroid drugs (steroids) mimic the action of the natural circulating glucocorticosteroids, cortisone and hydrocortisone (produced by the adrenal glands). These natural hormones are produced in response to stress, injury, or severe infection. Corticosteroids (such as hydrocortisone or dexamethasone) may be injected locally to reduce inflammation, particularly in the joints (such as in rheumatoid arthritis). In soft tissue conditions such as tennis elbow or tendonitis, where prior non-steroidal anti-inflammatory treatments have been unsuccessful, a small volume of corticosteroid may be injected to relieve inflammation and associated pain. Each joint should be treated no more than three times in one year.

3 **Compound analgesics contain simple analgesia and a low-dose opioid.**

A compound analgesic is a pain-relieving preparation with more than one active ingredient. This includes many of the stronger prescription analgesics. Common active ingredients used in compound analgesics include aspirin, paracetamol, and codeine. *Co-codamol 8/500* is the most commonly prescribed preparation; it contains 8 mg of codeine and 500 mg of paracetamol (thus the numbers are interpreted as top-line = opioid, bottom line = specific simple analgesic agent). Even this low dose of opioid is often sufficient to cause opioid-related side-effects (mainly constipation). Once readily available over the counter and in supermarkets, compound analgesics have become associated with substance abuse and their supply is now restricted as prescription-only medicines (POM) in the UK and many other countries.

4 **Patients on long-term corticosteroid treatment are at risk of serious side-effects.**

Side-effects of corticosteroid treatment are more likely when a patient is taking systemic medication or a high dose over an extended period. With inhaled corticosteroids or corticosteroids injected into a muscle or joint, the effects are targeted to one part of the body; therefore, side-effects tend to be limited to that specific region of the body. Long-term use of systemic or high-dose corticosteroids can cause hyperglycaemia and sodium retention, while potassium and calcium are lost via the kidneys. The adrenal glands cease to make the natural glucocorticosteroids and the body becomes reliant on the corticosteroid drugs for its supply of glucocorticosteroids. The hyperglycaemia may cause secondary diabetes, while the increased sodium in the blood will cause the kidneys to retain excess water, which increases overall blood volume and can lead to hypertension. The reduction in calcium can cause osteoporosis and increase the likelihood of a bone fracture. The gluconeogenesis (formation of glucose from non-carbohydrate sources namely amino acids and fats) can cause muscle deterioration and in children this may lead to growth retardation. Since the adrenal glands may stop producing natural glucocorticosteroids, patients must be weaned off long-term steroid treatment (usually over a period of about two months) to allow the body to recover its natural synthesis. Nurses should ensure that patients understand that if steroid treatment is stopped abruptly, the body can suffer a life-threatening steroidal (or adrenal) crisis due to the sudden insufficient levels of natural glucocorticosteroids.

5 **Antibacterial drugs target bacterial cells in the human body but do not harm human cells.**

For antibacterial (antibiotic) agents to be effective, they must kill bacterial cells but not harm human cells. To do this they specifically target components of bacterial cells that are not present in human cells, but since the structure of human cells and bacterial cells differs quite significantly, there are a number of potential targets that antibacterials can act upon to kill bacterial cells. Antibacterial drugs are usually divided into two groups: (1) bacteriostatic – meaning the drug inhibits the growth of the organism, which enables the body's immune system to recognize and destroy the bacterial colony; and (2) bactericidal – meaning the drug kills the bacteria. Antibacterial drugs that target the cell wall tend to be bactericidal in nature, while drugs that interfere with protein synthesis tend to be bacteriostatic (although they may have bactericidal properties at higher doses).

6 **The threadworm is a relatively common cause of helminth infection in the UK, especially in children.**

Threadworms (seatworms, pinworms) hatch and live primarily in the intestines. The eggs usually enter the body through the anus, nose or mouth via inhaled air or through the mouth on fingers that have touched a contaminated object. Symptoms of infection include anal itching and upset stomach. Treatment involves the whole household (irrespective of symptoms, due to their contagious nature) and includes rigorous hygiene and hand washing, together with a dose of mebendazole, which inhibits glucose uptake by the threadworm, leading to death of the pathogen within a few days. Since mebendazole kills the threadworms but not their eggs, it is important to prevent re-infection in the six weeks following treatment to stop re-infection. Generally threadworms do not cause serious complications.

7 | **Gram-positive bacteria will not absorb the purple-coloured Gram stain.**

Gram-negative bacteria do not absorb the Gram stain because they have a complex cell wall through which the stain cannot penetrate. The same principle applies to antibacterial treatment; certain antibacterial agents cannot penetrate the complex cell wall of a Gram-negative bacteria, thus the antibacterial agent will not be effective in treating a bacterial infection due to a Gram-negative bacteria. Gram-positive bacteria will absorb the purple Gram stain since their cell wall is structurally thinner and less complex; these bacteria are more susceptible to antibacterial drugs.

8 | **Broad-spectrum antibacterials should only be prescribed when the type of bacterial causing an infection is known.**

Broad-spectrum antibacterials are effective against a wide range of bacteria, including both Gram-positive and Gram-negative strains. This makes them useful when treating an infection when the bacterial cause has not been identified. For example, when a patient presents with the classic symptoms of meningitis, he or she should immediately receive a broad-spectrum antibacterial agent – usually benzylpenicillin or cefotaxime – to treat the infection, which is administered by IV to hasten the onset of action in treating the infection. Narrow-spectrum antibacterials target specific families of bacteria that tend to be either Gram-negative or Gram-positive.

MULTIPLE CHOICE

Correct answers identified in bold italics.

9 | **The recommended adult dose of oral paracetamol is:**

a) 0.25–0.5 g, no more than 2 g in 24 hours
b) 0.5–1.0 g, no more than 2 g in 24 hours
c) 0.25–0.5 g, no more than 4 g in 24 hours
d) *0.5–1.0 g, no more than 4 g in 24 hours*

The BNF currently recommends that paracetamol is administered to adults in doses of 0.5–1.0 g every 4–6 hours with no more than 4 g ingested in any 24-hour period. This is to prevent an overdose of paracetamol, which can cause liver damage. Paracetamol is quickly absorbed and serum levels peak within 30 minutes of administration. It has a relatively short half-life of about 2 hours, so it is eliminated quite quickly. It is widely used as an over-the-counter pain-relieving medicine but patients should be careful not to accidentally overdose on it, as it is also contained within a variety of cold and flu remedies to relieve symptoms of these illnesses. Retailers are prohibited from selling large quantities of paracetamol to limit the possibility of accidental overdose or fatal suicide attempts.

10 **Paracetamol may be described as:**

a) anti-inflammatory and non-steroidal
b) *non-anti-inflammatory and non-steroidal*
c) anti-inflammatory and steroidal
d) non-anti-inflammatory and steroidal

Paracetamol is widely used to relieve pain and fever in adults and children because it has analgesic and antipyretic (fever-lowering) properties; it does not have any anti-inflammatory properties. Its mechanism of action is not completely known but it does not target either the COX-1 or the COX-2 enzyme, so it has fewer undesirable GI side-effects commonly associated with the NSAIDs. Although it has relatively few side-effects, patients must be careful not to accidently overdose, as this can cause serious liver damage, even at two or three times the therapeutic dose.

11 **A major structural difference between bacterial and human cells is:**

a) *bacterial cells have a cell wall*
b) bacterial cells have no nucleus
c) bacterial cells have multiple nuclei
d) there are no differences

Human cells do not have a cell wall, they only have a cell membrane. Bacterial cells have a cell wall made up of peptidoglycan – this is unique to bacteria and this unique property is exploited in antibacterial drugs leaving human cells unharmed. The production of the peptidoglycan cell wall is dependent on an enzyme called transpeptidase (which is also unique to bacteria) and it is this enzyme that beta-lactam antibacterials target to kill bacteria. When the transpeptidase enzyme is inhibited, the bacterial cell wall synthesis is disrupted, which compromises the integrity of the bacterial cell wall causing the bacteria to lyse and die.

12 **Which of the following types of antibacterials is not a part of the beta-lactam family?**

a) penicillins
b) carbapenems
c) cephalosporins
d) *tetracyclines*

The beta-lactam family of antibacterials are grouped together because they have a similar chemical structure – a 'ring' shape – that is essential to the pharmacological activity of these drugs. The penicillins, carbapenems, and cephalosporins all have a beta-lactam ring and so are part of the beta-lactam family. Tetracyclines belong to a different class of antibacterials that inhibit protein synthesis in bacteria by targeting the ribosomes of bacterial cells, since they have a slightly different structure from human ribosomes. These ribosome-targeting antibacterials are bacteriostatic in nature. Tetracyclines are widely used in the treatment of urinary tract infections (UTIs) and respiratory tract infections (RTIs), and are also used to treat chlamydia and bacterial meningitis.

13 **The most serious side-effect associated with penicillin is:**

a) nausea and vomiting   b) diarrhoea

c) *anaphylaxis*   d) drowsiness

As many as 10% of people are believed to be hypersensitive to penicillin. These patients can experience a mild hypersensitivity reaction such as a rash or headache but in a rare number of cases this reaction can be severe, causing anaphylaxis, which can be fatal. Anaphylaxis (or anaphylactic shock) is a severe, potentially life-threatening, allergic reaction that can affect many of the systems of the body, including the airways, breathing, and blood circulation. If anaphylaxis is suspected, it should be treated as a medical emergency because of the rapid onset of these serious symptoms. The patient should be administered adrenaline as quickly as possible to raise blood pressure, relieve breathing difficulties, and reduce swelling. Hypersensitivity is more likely to occur in individuals who suffer from other allergies. In cases where a minor localized rash develops or the rash develops more than 72 hours after administration of penicillin, these reactions may not be specifically attributable to penicillin and these patients should not be prohibited from taking penicillin to treat serious infections. Other beta-lactam antibacterials are generally safe to use in these patients.

14 **Which of the following antibacterials may be used in patients who are penicillin-hypersensitive?**

a) erythromycin   b) amoxicillin   c) benzylpenicillin   d) co-amoxiclav

Patients who are known to be penicillin-hypersensitive should not be prescribed any form of penicillin or penicillin-derivative such as amoxicillin, benzylpenicillin or co-amoxiclav, since the hypersensitivity is due to the beta-lactam structure of penicillin. They may also react to the other beta-lactam antibacterials (cephalosporins and carbapenams), since they are structurally similar to penicillins. When such patients require antibacterial treatment they are usually prescribed erythromycin, which belongs to the macrolide antibacterial family but has a similar antibacterial spectrum to that of penicillin.

15 **Which of the following ribosome-targeting antibacterials is not well absorbed when administered orally?**

a) tetracyclines

b) aminoglycosides

c) chloramphenicol

d) erythromycin

The aminoglycosides include gentamycin and neomycin. None of the group is well absorbed when administered orally, thus they are usually administered by IV or IM injection. Caution is advised when administering any aminoglycoside to patients with renal problems, as they can damage the nephrons of the kidneys, although this can usually be reversed by immediately stopping the drug. They are also known to irreversibly damage the inner ear.

16 **This group of antibacterial agents interferes with folic acid synthesis by bacteria:**

a) fluoroquinolones

b) beta-lactams

c) tetracyclines

d) sulphonamides

The sulphonamides inhibit the action of para-aminobenzoic acid (PABA), which is essential for the production of folic acid by bacterial cells (human cells can absorb folic acid from the diet, whereas bacterial cells must synthesize it). In the absence of PABA, folic acid is not produced and cell replication is inhibited (therefore sulphonamides are bacteriostatic in nature). Trimethoprim is a well-known sulphonamide that is sometimes used to treat UTIs, acute and chronic bronchitis, and certain types of bacterial pneumonia. However, the use of sulphonamides has decreased due to increased bacterial resistance and the availability of new, less toxic antibacterial drugs.

17 **Which of the following type of drugs is not considered part of the 'analgesic ladder'?**

a) strong opioids

b) mild opioids

c) beta$_2$ agonists

d) non-opioids

Beta$_2$ agonists are bronchodilator drugs commonly used in the treatment of asthma and certain forms of COPD (see Chapter 8); they do not offer any form of pain relief and are not part of the analgesic ladder. The analgesic (or pain) ladder was devised by the World Health Organization (WHO) (see Figure 2.1) for the successful drug management of cancer pain. It describes a stepwise approach to the pharmacological management of pain and it is applicable to the management of other types of pain such as post-operative pain. It is based on the principle that pain management should start at the first step and then proceed up the ladder if pain is still present. The pain medications range from over-the-counter drugs that have minimal side-effects, such as paracetamol or NSAIDs at the first step, proceeding to weak/mild opioids, such as codeine (which may be administered in combination with a non-opioid) at the second step, and eventually proceeding to powerful opioids, such as morphine (which, again, may be administered in combination

Figure 2.1 The three-step analgesic ladder (adapted from the World Health Organization's Three-Step Analgesic Ladder)

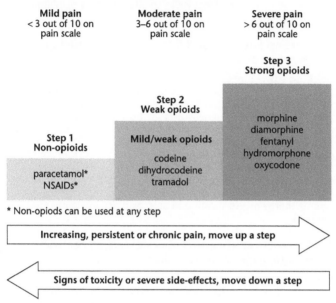

* Non-opiods can be used at any step

with a non-opioid), at the third step. Its success relies on selecting the appropriate drug at the correct dosage and balancing efficacy against adverse effects. Other drugs such as local anesthetics and certain antidepressants may also be used to relieve pain.

FILL IN THE BLANKS

18 ***Corticosteroids*** **are anti-inflammatory drugs that reduce inflammation and suppress immune responses.**

The anti-inflammatory properties associated with corticosteroid drugs are thought to be due to their combined action on the immune cells and chemicals associated with the inflammatory response. This gives them powerful anti-inflammatory and immunosuppressive properties that inhibit the inflammatory response and influence tissue healing and repair. They are used for a wide range of conditions, including autoimmune disorders (such as rheumatoid arthritis and Crohn's disease), allergic/hypersensitivity reactions (such as asthma and hay fever), and to prevent organ transplant rejection. However, this wide-ranging anti-inflammatory and immunosuppressive activity can also make a patient more susceptible to infection (because their immune system is compromised), it can mask infections, and decreases the healing potential of tissues. Corticosteroids may be administered locally via inhalation, cream, ointment or local injection or they may be delivered systemically.

19 **Selective cyclooxygenase-2 inhibitors may be used to treat *chronic inflammatory* diseases.**

Selective COX-2 inhibitors, such as etoricoxib and celecoxib, have a high specificity for COX-2. At low concentrations, these drugs do not inhibit the action of COX-1, so the production of prostaglandins associated with normal tissue homeostasis is not affected, which reduces the undesirable side-effects associated with the non-selective NSAIDs. The reduction in GI side-effects makes selective COX-2 inhibitors more desirable for long-term use in chronic inflammatory conditions such as Crohn's disease or rheumatoid arthritis. Unfortunately, a number of adverse effects, including liver toxicity and coronary heart disease, have been associated with their use and a number of these drugs have been withdrawn (etoricoxib and celecoxib are currently still licensed in the UK).

20 **Antibacterials, antifungals, antiprotozoals, and antivirals all belong to the *antimicrobial* family of drugs.**

For any antimicrobial drug to be effective, it must be able to kill or limit the growth of the infecting pathogen (microorganism) without severely affecting human cells. This is known as selective toxicity. For bacteria, differences in structural components (such as the cell wall, minor differences in the ribosomes and DNA replication) are usually the targets for antimicrobial drugs. Finding successful antimicrobial agents that target and kill other pathogens such as fungi, protozoa, and helminths, along with pathogens that act as intracellular parasites (viruses and certain bacteria) is much more difficult, since these pathogens are structurally more similar to human cells and can enter human cells, often using the human cell's own enzymes in their metabolic processes, to grow and replicate. The cells of fungal pathogens differ only slightly in their cell membranes, which contain a molecule called ergosterol (rather than cholesterol in human cell membranes). Antifungal drugs, such as amphotericin, bind to ergosterol and disrupt the cell membrane, causing cell lysis and death of the fungal pathogen. Viruses can only replicate once inside a host cell, which makes them very difficult to treat. Some treatments, such as aciclovir (which targets the *Herpes* virus), have been developed that target proteins unique to viruses but the main form of defence against viral infection is vaccination, which prepares the human immune system to defend itself against certain viruses.

21 **Toxoplasmosis and trichomoniasis are the most common *protozoal* infections in the UK.**

Diseases caused by protozoa tend to be found in more tropical regions of the world and so are relatively uncommon in the UK. Toxoplasmosis is an infection transmitted from animals such as cats and rabbits; pregnant women and immunocompromised patients are particularly susceptible to it. Trichomoniasis is a relatively common sexually transmitted infection that is treated with the antibacterial metronidazole. Malaria is also a protozoal infection, although it is usually contracted in other parts of the world. When people in the UK contract malaria, it is often after they have been abroad to an at-risk region and not taken the correct prophylactic antimalarial treatments or not followed the instructions for prophylactic treatment accurately.

22 *Beta-lactamase* **is an enzyme produced by resistant bacteria that makes antibacterial drugs ineffective.**

Bacteria have many ways of overcoming the effects of antibacterial drugs and developing resistance. The most effective means is the development of bacteria capable of producing an enzyme called beta-lactamase that denatures (breaks) the beta-lactam ring of the relevant antibiotics, rendering the drugs ineffective. To overcome bacterial resistance due to beta-lactamase-producing bacteria such as strains of *Escherichia coli* or *Staphylococcus aureus*, co-amoxiclav may be prescribed. This is a combination of amoxicillin and clavulanic acid. Although clavulanic acid is not an antibacterial agent, it is similar in structure to penicillin. It inhibits the beta-lactamase enzyme, allowing the amoxicillin to act on the bacteria and destroy it. Co-amoxiclav is usually prescribed in the format x/y where x = strength of amoxicillin in milligrams and y = strength of clavulanic acid in milligrams, for example, *co-amoxiclav 250/125* = amoxicillin 250 mg and clavulanic acid 125 mg.

23 *Tetracyclines* **bind to a number of ions and metals, which inhibits their absorption.**

Tetracyclines are usually taken orally before meals, since they are best absorbed on an empty stomach. Patients should be advised not to take oral tetracyclines with milk as the drug binds to calcium, which prevents its absorption in the GI tract. The drug also binds to magnesium, aluminium, and iron, so medicines containing these metals should be avoided while taking tetracyclines. Gastrointestinal disturbance is the most common side-effect with the tetracyclines, which is due to their ability to disturb the balance of normal intestinal flora. Prolonged treatment with tetracyclines, particularly in children, can interfere with teeth and bone formation because of their ability to bind with calcium. For this reason, they should also be avoided during pregnancy.

24 **The** *fluoroquinolone* **family of antibacterials inhibits DNA replication and protein synthesis.**

The fluoroquinolones (or quinolones) are a relatively new group of broad-spectrum antibacterials that inhibit the topoisomerase II enzyme involved in DNA replication, thus bacterial cells cannot replicate their DNA. The most common drug in this group is ciprofloxacin, which is used to treat certain STIs such as chlamydia and gonorrhoea. It is well absorbed when administered orally but should not be taken with antacids since it binds to metals, which prevents its absorption in the GI tract.

25 ***Opioids* produce analgesia by acting on the central nervous system.**

Opioid analgesics are drugs that exert their pain-relieving activity by acting as agonists at opioid receptors and blocking the transmission of pain signals across the synapse of neurones. These receptors are widespread throughout the central nervous system. Morphine, codeine, pethidine, tramadol, fentanyl, and diamorphine are part of the opioid family of analgesic medicines. Each opioid drug has its own specific onset of action, duration of effect, and associated side-effects. Morphine is generally considered the most useful opioid for managing severe pain. Due to their strong effects on the nervous system, opioids have a number of side-effects, including nausea and vomiting (especially after initial administration) and a decrease in gastric motility (particularly with codeine), which can cause constipation or suppression of the respiratory system (this is why an overdose of morphine may be fatal). Local anaesthetics act peripherally while NSAIDs have effects on both the central and peripheral nervous systems.

Figure 2.2 Drugs associated with infection

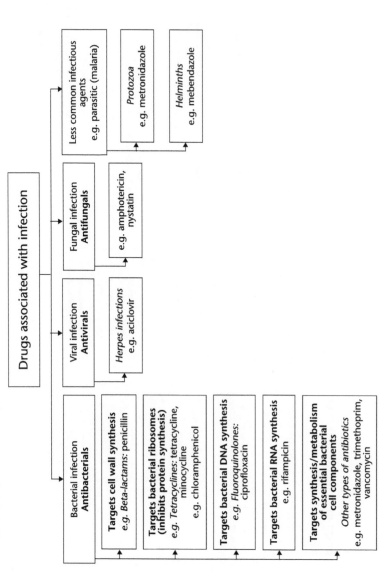

Figure 2.3 Drugs used for inflammation and/or pain management

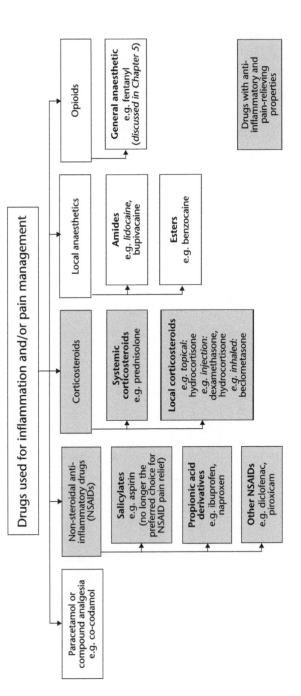

3 Drugs and the integumentary system

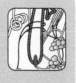

INTRODUCTION

The integumentary system comprises a number of organs that include the skin and its associated accessory structures – hair, nails, glands, and nerve endings. As an organ system, the integument has a variety of functions: to waterproof, cushion, and protect the deeper tissues; assist in the excretion of waste; and help regulate body temperature. It is also the site for attachment of sensory receptors involved in the detection of pain, sensation, pressure and temperature, and it absorbs vitamin D from ultraviolet (UV) light.

The external location of the skin and its accessory structures makes it vulnerable to infection, trauma, and certain environmental insults, but similarly allows for the easy application of medicines that may be used to treat not only conditions of the skin, but those of other body systems.

Skin conditions can trigger a range of symptoms including a rash, pain, stinging, and itching. However, the skin can also display symptoms of systemic illness such as liver or endocrine disorders and childhood illnesses such as chicken pox and measles.

Pharmacological treatments administered via the skin must be fat- and water-soluble to be absorbed across the skin. The nurse should be aware that many types of medication used to treat disorders of other tissues or organs can cause hypersensitivity of the skin, often making skin more sensitive to UV light or altering pigmentation. Often patients may attempt to treat such reactions without seeking medical advice, which can exacerbate the reaction.

Useful resources

Nurses! Test Yourself in Anatomy and Physiology
Chapter 3

Nurses! Test Yourself in Pathophysiology
Chapter 3

Further Essentials of Pharmacology for Nurses
Chapter 8

TRUE OR FALSE?

Are the following statements true or false?

1 Topical corticosteroids have anti-inflammatory and antipruritic properties.

2 Tacrolimus is useful for the treatment of severe eczema (atopic dermatitis).

3 Head lice are treated with antibiotic lotions.

4 Topical corticosteroids are contra-indicated in rosacea.

5 Preparations containing coal tar are useful in the treatment of plaque psoriasis.

6 Topical antibacterial preparations of erythromycin and clindamycin are generally effective for mild inflammatory acne.

7 Drug-induced photosensitivity is not a side-effect of drugs.

8 Retapamulin is effective in treating superficial skin infections caused by MRSA.

9   Compound topical preparations containing an imidazole and a mild corticosteroid may be required to treat inflammatory skin conditions with fungal infections.

10   Benzyl benzoate is one of the most effective treatments for head lice.

MULTIPLE CHOICE

Identify one correct answer for each of the following.

11 Solutions containing cetrimide may be used to treat:

    a) middle ear infections

    b) mild burns

    c) scabies

    d) urticaria

12 Emollients are typically used on skin to:

    a) cleanse

    b) dehydrate

    c) hydrate

    d) disinfect

13 Azaleic acid is primarily used to treat:

    a) rosacea

    b) inflammatory acne

    c) cellulitis

    d) parasitic infestations of the skin

14 Psoriasis can be treated with:

    a) both topical and systemic preparations

    b) systemic preparations only

    c) topical preparations only

    d) phototherapy only

15 The most effective pharmacological treatment for contact dermatitis involves the use of:

a) broad-spectrum antibiotics

b) scabicides

c) topical corticosteroids

d) kerolytics

16 Which of the following tetracycline antibiotics has the broadest spectrum of antimicrobial activity?

a) tetracycline

b) doxycycline

c) lymecycline

d) minocycline

FILL IN THE BLANKS

Fill in the blanks in each statement using the options in the box below.
Not all of them are required, so choose carefully!

lidocaine	nappy rash
salicylic acid	emollient
sun protection	weeping eczema
antibacterial	ultraviolet
capsaicin	

17 An _____ can be useful when treating pruritus associated with dry skin.

18 The _____ _____ factor given on the packaging of sunscreen preparations provides guidance on protection against U V B.

19 _____ _____ is a type of contact dermatitis best treated with a barrier cream preparation.

20 Cellulitis requires systemic _____ treatment.

21 _____ _____ is useful for the removal of corns and calluses.

22 _____ cream or ointment may be used to relieve deep muscle pain or nervous system pain.

MATCH THE TERMS

Match each of the following skin medications with the listed pharmacological functions:

A. antipruritic

B. local anaesthetic

C. corticosteroid

D. antiseptic

E. antiparasitic

F. emollient

G. topical antibacterial

H. keratolytic

I. antineoplastic agent

J. antifungal

| 23 | Neomycin | 28 | Lidocaine |

| 24 | Fluorouracil | 29 | Nystatin cream |

| 25 | Salicylic acid | 30 | Aqueous cream |

| 26 | Betamethasone | 31 | Chlorhexidine |

| 27 | Calamine | 32 | Malathion |

ANSWERS

TRUE OR FALSE

1 **Topical corticosteroids have anti-inflammatory and antipruritic properties.**

Topical corticosteroids (steroids) are useful in the treatment of many inflammatory and pruritic (itching) skin conditions such as eczema, psoriasis, and atopic dermatitis. However, corticosteroid treatment is not curative and the effects of this type of drug are limited by the duration of its use, thus recurrence or exacerbations of the condition often occur when treatment is discontinued. In general, a low-dose corticosteroid should be used where possible and treatment discontinued as soon as the condition improves, since the incidence of side-effects associated with topical corticosteroids (such as thinning of the skin, altered pigmentation, and burning of the skin) increases with higher concentrations and prolonged use.

2 **Tacrolimus is useful for the treatment of severe eczema (atopic dermatitis).**

Tacrolimus is a prescription-only, non-steroidal immunosuppressant that may also be used to prevent organ rejection. It may be used in the treatment of moderate-to-severe eczema when more conventional first-line treatments (such as emollients and corticosteroids) have been unsuccessful. It reduces inflammation and should be used with lots of emollient but not under wet wraps. It is also used to treat psoriasis. A burning sensation of the skin is a common side-effect of tacrolimus and exposure to sunlight should be limited. Continuous, long-term treatment should be avoided.

3 **Head lice are treated with antibiotic lotions.**

Head lice are a parasitic infection (as are crab lice and scabies) that can be treated with parasiticidal preparations – preferably in liquid or lotion formulations for head lice treatment. Malathion and the pyrethroid phenothrin are frequently prescribed to treat head lice. Dimeticone may be used if resistance is suspected, although it is less effective against lice eggs. Benzyl benzoate may be used but is less effective. Head lice can be physically eradicated by thoroughly combing wet hair with a detection comb. Permethrin is not suitable for treating head lice due to its formulation. For treatment of crab lice (elsewhere on the body), malathion, phenothrin, and permethrin can be used.

4 **Topical corticosteroids are contra-indicated in rosacea.**

Although topical corticosteroids, such as hydrocortisone, are frequently used to treat inflammatory conditions of the skin (for example, eczema), they are contra-indicated in the treatment of rosacea as they can exacerbate ulcerated or infected pustules. Treatment is usually with metronidazole or topical azelaic acid. The redness associated with rosacea can be concealed with a camouflage cream.

5 | **Preparations containing coal tar are useful in the treatment of plaque psoriasis.**

The aim of treatment for psoriasis is to normalize the rate of production of skin cells, improve hydration of the skin, and reduce the associated inflammation. Non-emulsifying ointments with appropriate active ingredients added are commonly used to treat chronic dry skin conditions like psoriasis. Coal tar is an anti-inflammatory, antimitotic agent and is still the preferred treatment for psoriasis, since it has fewer side-effects. A liquid preparation may be added to bath water when treating psoriasis.

6 | **Topical antibacterial preparations of erythromycin and clindamycin are generally effective for mild inflammatory acne.**

Topical antibacterial preparations such as erythromycin and clindamycin are usually effective for mild inflammatory acne, although they may cause irritation to the skin and in certain cases sensitization may occur. For many patients with mild-to-moderate inflammatory acne, topical antibacterial preparations may be no more effective than topical non-antibiotic antimicrobials such as benzoyl peroxide or azelaic acid, or tretinoin (a topical retinoid). Some patients report less local irritation with azelaic acid medicines than benzoyl peroxide. Given the increase in bacterial resistance to antibiotics, the latter treatments are often preferable as first-line treatments for acne before considering topical antibacterials. If topical preparations fail to eradicate the acne, then oral options may be recommended.

7 | **Drug-induced photosensitivity is not a side-effect of drugs.**

Many common medications (both topical and systemic preparations) can cause a photosensitive reaction of the skin when a patient is exposed to sunlight during treatment. Photosensitivity is due to the combined effects of light and the medication – each alone will not trigger photosensitivity. Photosensitivity reactions can be either phototoxic or photoallergic. Phototoxic reactions are more common and can develop after a lot of exposure to both light and drug; it appears as severe sunburn only over the area exposed to the light and drug. Photoallergic reactions are less common and tend to be due to an immune response to a light-activated compound in the medication; symptoms resemble contact dermatitis over the exposed area, although the rash may spread to non-exposed areas. Many drugs, such as the antibiotic tetracycline, the NSAID ibuprofen, and the diuretic furosemide, will trigger phototoxic photosensitivity reactions if exposure to light is prolonged. Fewer medications trigger photoallergic reactions, but include certain hypoglycaemics, statins, and antipsychotic drugs. Topical corticosteroids may be administered to relieve drug-induced photosensitivity, while systemic corticosteroids should only be used in severe cases.

8 **Retapamulin is effective in treating superficial skin infections caused by MRSA.**

Retapamulin is a topical antibacterial preparation effective in the treatment of superficial skin infections, such as impetigo, caused by certain strains of *Staphylococcal* and *Streptococcal* bacteria that are resistant to first-line treatment (although in Scotland it is not recommended for treatment of superficial skin infections). It is not effective against MRSA and therefore should not be used where MRSA infection is suspected. If MRSA is suspected in superficial skin infections, a tetracycline can be used alone or in combination with sodium fusidate or rifampicin; alternatively, clindamycin may be used alone. For severe skin infections caused by MRSA, a glycopeptide such as vancomycin is recommended.

9 **Compound topical preparations containing an imidazole and a mild corticosteroid may be required to treat inflammatory skin conditions with fungal infections.**

Candidal intertrigo is an example of an inflammatory skin condition where a fungal infection is also present. It can be thought of as 'thrush' of the skinfolds (and is also known as infected sweat rash or fungal sweat rash). It is characterized by a sore, itchy rash on the skin where sweat is trapped and is therefore common in the folds of the skin where skin may chafe. It is a problem experienced by patients who are immobile or overweight and in diabetic patients. To treat this type of infection a compound preparation may be prescribed containing a topical antifungal agent such as the imidazole clotrimazole to treat the fungal infection, in combination with an anti-inflammatory such as the corticosteroid hydrocortisone to treat the rash. These agents are available as compound preparations of 1% hydrocortisone, 1% clotrimazole. When the inflammation clears, it may be necessary to continue the antifungal treatment alone for a few days longer.

10 **Benzyl benzoate is one of the most effective treatments for head lice.**

Benzyl benzoate is licensed for the treatment of head lice but is much less effective than malathion and dimeticone, which are more commonly used to treat infestations. Benzyl benzoate may act as an irritant and should not be used when treating children. Head lice should be treated using topical lotions (shampoos are often too dilute to be effective) and thorough combing of the hair with a detection comb. To be effective, a course of treatment usually requires two applications seven days apart to ensure eradication of all lice and eggs.

MULTIPLE CHOICE

Correct answers identified in bold italics.

11 Solutions containing cetrimide may be used to treat:

a) middle ear infections *b) mild burns* c) scabies d) urticaria

Cetrimide is a mild antiseptic that may be used to prevent infections from cuts, grazes, minor burns, minor scalds, minor wounds, and minor abrasions. It may be used in children, adults, and the elderly.

12 Emollients are typically used on skin to:

a) cleanse b) dehydrate *c) hydrate* d) disinfect

Emollients are topical treatments that reduce water loss from the outer layer of skin (epidermis) by covering it with a protective film that allows damaged cells on the skin's surface to repair themselves. These treatments are also known as moisturizers and come in several forms, including soap substitutes, bath oils, moisturizing creams, and ointments. In addition to helping the skin retain water, emollients can also be used to moisturize dry skin, ease itching, soften cracks, and can allow other topical treatments to enter the skin.

13 Azelaic acid is primarily used to treat:

a) rosacea   *b) inflammatory acne*
c) cellulitis   d) parasitic infestations of the skin

Azelaic acid has antimicrobial properties and is primarily used to treat mild-to-moderate acne by killing the bacteria that infect pores, forming lesions and reducing the production of keratin (which is thought to contribute to the development of acne). It is available as a gel or a cream and may be used as an alternative to a benzyl peroxide preparation for acne of the face, as some patients report less local irritation with azelaic acid than benzyl peroxide. Azelaic acid can also be used in the treatment of rosacea and for certain skin pigmentation disorders.

14 Psoriasis can be treated with:

a) both topical and systemic preparations

b) systemic preparations only

c) topical preparations only

d) phototherapy only

Treatment of psoriasis depends on the type, severity, and location of the inflammation. First-line treatment for mild cases of psoriasis involves topical medications such as emollients and skin softeners. Topical drugs such as vitamin D (calcitriol) and its analogues (calcipotriol and tacalcitol) are often used to treat plaque psoriasis, although these can cause local irritation such as itching, erythema, and paraesthesia. Coal tar preparations may be used to treat chronic plaque psoriasis due to its anti-inflammatory and antiscaling properties; it is not usually harmful to normal skin and tar preparations are available for bathing. Topical corticosteroids are not usually recommended for long-term use, although they may be used as short-term treatment of a specific area such as the face. Phototherapy (in the form of ultraviolet B (UVB) radiation) is sometimes used to treat moderately severe psoriasis that does not respond well to topical treatments, although it can exacerbate inflammatory psoriasis. If psoriasis is severe, systemic medication that targets the immune system may be employed such as methotrexate or ciclosporin. Use of these preparations requires specialist supervision (sometimes in hospital).

15 **The most effective pharmacological treatment for contact dermatitis involves the use of:**

a) broad-spectrum antibiotics

b) scabicides

c) *topical corticosteroids*

d) kerolytics

The most effective means of treating contact dermatitis is to avoid contact with the allergen or irritant. Topical corticosteroid medications are most useful in the treatment of severe contact dermatitis. There are many formulations of corticosteroids in a range of different potencies. Creams, lotions, and gels are available that allow the active steroid to penetrate deep into the skin layers for relief of local inflammation, burning, and itching. Long-term use of corticosteroids is not recommended due to the potential for irritation, redness, and thinning of mucous membranes.

16 **Which of the following tetracycline antibiotics has the broadest spectrum of antimicrobial activity?**

a) tetracycline b) doxycycline c) lymecycline **d)** *minocycline*

The tetracyclines are a family of broad-spectrum antibiotics, most of which do not vary greatly in their antimicrobial activity except for minocycline, which has a broader spectrum of activity. Minocycline can be used to treat irreversible pigmentation and lupus-erythematosus-like syndrome. The use of tetracyclines has decreased due to the rise of bacterial resistance yet they are still the treatment of choice for certain infections such as chlamydia and are used in the treatment of some MRSA infections. They are also used to treat certain respiratory infections caused by mycoplasma and may be prescribed to treat acne.

FILL IN THE BLANKS

17 An *emollient* can be useful when treating pruritus associated with dry skin.

Pruritus (itching) may be caused by several types of systemic disease, as a result of skin disease, or as a side-effect of opioid analgesics. Where possible the underlying cause should be addressed to reduce the symptom. However, an emollient may be applied if the pruritus is associated with dry skin, as it will soothe and hydrate the affected area.

18 The *sun protection* factor given on the packaging of sunscreen preparations provides guidance on protection against UVB.

Ultraviolet radiation emitted by the sun produces two types of wavelengths that can damage skin. The long ultraviolet A (UVA) wavelengths can cause photosensitivity reactions and photodermatoses, while the medium ultraviolet B (UVB) wavelengths cause sunburn. The sun protection factor (SPF) rating of a sunscreen indicates the degree of protection offered against UVB rays by the formulation. For example, a product with a SPF rating of 15 should protect sun-exposed skin from burning for 15 times longer that unprotected skin. Protection against UVA rays is indicated by a star rating, but many sunscreen preparations offer little or no protection against UVA rays. The most effective UVA sunscreen preparations are those that contain reflective compounds such as titanium dioxide; a number of such formulations are available over-the-counter or on prescription.

19 *Nappy rash* is a type of contact dermatitis best treated with a barrier cream preparation.

Nappy rash is a common type of dermatitis that can usually be controlled by barrier creams that reduce the contact of the baby's skin with urine and faeces. Zinc cream, zinc oxide ointment, and petroleum jelly are all suitable barrier creams. In mild cases, it is suggested that the baby's nappy be left off for as long as possible between changes or during sleep. Avoid bathing baby too frequently, as this may dry out the skin and promote a more severe nappy rash.

20 Cellulitis requires systemic *antibacterial* treatment.

Cellulitis is an infection of the dermis and subcutaneous layers of the skin. It is characterized by hot, red, painful, and swollen areas of skin, most often occurring on the legs or feet, although it can present anywhere on the body. Cellultis is most commonly caused by *Staphylococcal* bacteria, although *Streptococci* are also known to trigger the infection. First-line treatment is usually with a seven-day course of the penicillin flucloxacillin, which is often sufficient to eradicate mild cellulitis caused by *Staphylococcal* bacteria. In more severe cases, a combination of oral flucloxacillin and phenoxymethylpenicillin (penicillin V) should be prescribed; if *Streptococcal* infection is diagnosed, flucloxacillin should be discontinued. Patients who are penicillin-allergic should be treated with erythromycin alone. Patients should be advised to rest, drink lots of water, and elevate the affected leg (if appropriate); paracetamol or ibuprofen may also be prescribed to reduce pain, fever, and swelling. Hospital admission for IV antibiotic treatment may be required if a patient fails to respond to oral antibiotics or if the infection spreads – in this situation, urgent medical attention should be sought, as a secondary infection may develop into septicaemia.

21 _**Salicylic acid**_ **is useful for the removal of corns and calluses.**

Corns and calluses arise when the stratum corneum of the epidermis becomes hard and thickened due to friction or pressure, and usually occur on the foot. The thickened skin may be treated with a salicylic acid preparation that softens thickened skin, making it easier to remove. The thickened skin can also be carefully removed with a scalpel. A wide range of salicylic acid treatments are available over-the-counter, although care should be taken not to apply the treatment to the normal skin surrounding the corn or callus because the treatment may damage normal skin since it is thinner.

22 _**Capsaicin**_ **cream or ointment may be used to relieve deep muscle pain or nervous system pain.**

Capsaicin is a natural ingredient found in chilli peppers that gives them their hot, spicy characteristic; it is used as a topical analgesic for pain relief in certain conditions. When first applied, a capsaicin preparation may cause a transient burning sensation that usually subsides. Capsaicin is thought to relieve pain by blocking pain receptors, which prevents the communication of pain signals between the central nervous system (CNS) (brain and spinal cord) and other parts of the body. Capsaicin is used topically to relieve muscle pain, joint pain, rheumatoid arthritis, neuralgia (pain associated with shingles), and diabetic neuropathy. Patients should be advised to thoroughly wash hands immediately after application (or 30 minutes after use if application is to the hands) and to avoid a hot bath or shower immediately before or after use, as the hot water may exacerbate any initial burning sensation.

MATCH THE TERMS

23	Neomycin	**G.** topical antibacterial
24	Fluorouracil	**I.** antineoplastic agent
25	Salicylic acid	**H.** keratolytic
26	Betamethasone	**C.** corticosteroid
27	Calamine	**A.** antipruritic
28	Lidocaine	**B.** local anaesthetic
29	Nystatin cream	**J.** antifungal
30	Aqueous cream	**F.** emollient
31	Chlorhexidine	**D.** antiseptic
32	Malathion	**E.** antiparasitic

Figure 3.1 Drugs used to treat common skin conditions

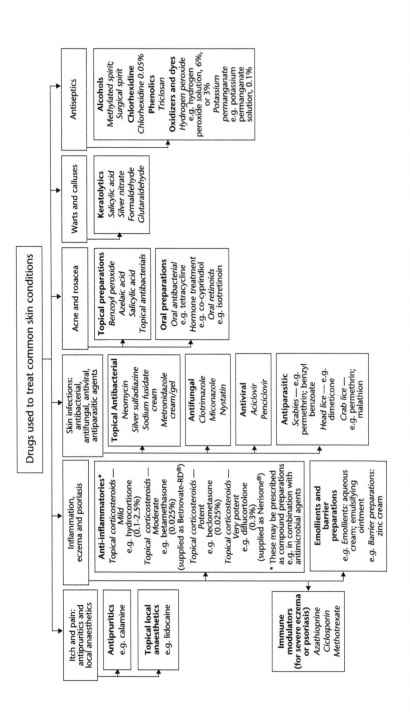

4 Drugs and the musculoskeletal system

INTRODUCTION

The musculoskeletal system consists of the skeletal system (made up of bones and joints of the axial and appendicular skeletons) and three types of muscle tissue – smooth, skeletal, and cardiac. The main functions of the system include support, movement, and protection of the body together with endocrine regulation, erythropoiesis, and storage of vital minerals.

Diseases and disorders of the musculoskeletal system can be acute (such as sprains and fractures), chronic (such as rheumatoid arthritis) or life-threatening (such as spinal injuries or multiple sclerosis). Treating acute disorders mainly involves immobilizing the affected limb, reducing swelling, and controlling pain. The treatment of chronic musculoskeletal disorders aims to control symptoms and slow progression by preventing joint damage.

Management of pain and inflammation is an important aspect of nursing care when treating disorders of the musculoskeletal system. Many of the drugs used in the treatment of chronic musculoskeletal disorders have side-effects that require clinical and laboratory monitoring to preserve mobility and quality of life for as long as possible. Patients should also be advised on the non-pharmacological management of their condition such as the importance of diet, exercise, and rest.

Useful resources

Nurses! Test Yourself in Anatomy and Physiology
Chapter 4

Nurses! Test Yourself in Pathophysiology
Chapter 4

Drug groups affecting the musculoskeletal system
http://www.patient.co.uk/leaflets/drug_groups_primarily_affecting_the_musculoskeletal_system.htm

TRUE OR FALSE?

Are the following statements true or false?

| 1 | The antimalarial hydroxychloroquine can be used to alleviate the symptoms of rheumatoid arthritis.

| 2 | A topical NSAID should be used as first-line treatment for the relief of pain in osteoarthritis and soft tissue disorders.

| 3 | Disease-modifying antirheumatic drugs (DMARDs) have an immediate therapeutic response.

| 4 | Skeletal muscle relaxants should be prescribed to treat spasm associated with minor injuries.

| 5 | Anticholinesterases reduce neuromuscular transmission in myasthenia gravis.

MULTIPLE CHOICE

Identify one correct answer for each of the following.

6 Which of the following does not describe a mechanism of action for antigout drugs?

a) drugs that act on the joint

b) drugs that act on the GI system

c) drugs that reduce uric acid synthesis

d) drugs that increase the excretion of uric acid by the kidneys

7 Local corticosteroid injection is not recommended as a treatment for:

a) rheumatoid arthritis

b) tennis elbow

c) carpal tunnel syndrome

d) inflammation of the Achilles tendon

8 Which of the following compounds may be used in second-line anti-arthritic treatments?

a) gold

b) silver

c) mercury

d) carbon dioxide

9 Cannabis extract is licensed as a treatment for which musculoskeletal disorder?

a) spinal cord injuries

b) nocturnal cramp

c) multiple sclerosis

d) osteomyelitis

10 Which of the following is considered first-line treatment for pain associated with osteoarthritis and soft tissues disorders?

a) NSAIDs

b) mild opioids

c) moderate opioids

d) paracetamol

FILL IN THE BLANKS

Fill in the blanks in each statement using the options in the box below.
Not all of them are required, so choose carefully!

---

rheumatoid arthritis	cyclosporin
atropine	NSAID
DMARD	hyaluronidase
azothioprine	myasthenia gravis

11 _____ is an immunosuppressant that may be used to treat severe, progressive rheumatoid arthritis.

12 The enzyme _____ can be used to make tissues more permeable to injected fluids.

13 _____ may be classified as a disease-modifying antirheumatic drug (DMARD).

14 Pyridostigmine bromide is used in the treatment of _____ _____.

15 Diclofenac is an _____ drug used to treat pain and inflammation associated with rheumatic disorders.

MATCH THE TERMS

Match each of the following agents with the listed pharmacological functions:

A. DMARD   D. uric acid lowering agent

B. corticosteroid   E. NSAID

C. anticholinesterase   F. skeletal muscle relaxant

16 Prednisolone   **19** Cyclosporin

17 Diclofenac   **20** Allopurinol

18 Diazepam   **21** Pyridostigmine bromide

ANSWERS

TRUE OR FALSE?

1 **The antimalarial hydroxychloroquine can be used to alleviate the symptoms of rheumatoid arthritis**

Antimalarial drugs such as hydroxychloroquine may be prescribed to alleviate moderate inflammatory symptoms of rheumatoid arthritis, although the mechanism of action is not understood. It is also used in the treatment of juvenile arthritis. Chloroquine is prescribed less frequently and usually only when other drugs have failed. Although rare when the drugs are used within the recommended doses, an adverse effect with this form of treatment is eye damage, which may or may not be irreversible, so regular ophthalmological monitoring for ocular toxicity is required. If visual or retinal changes are detected, hydroxychloroquine (or chloroquine) should not be prescribed. In older adults, it can be difficult to differentiate between age-induced and drug-induced retinopathy.

2 **A topical NSAID should be used as first-line treatment for the relief of pain in osteoarthritis and soft tissue disorders**

For osteoarthritis and other associated soft tissue disorders, paracetamol is indicated for the initial relief of pain. However, the medication may be required to be taken regularly for extended periods of time. A topical NSAID may be considered in moderate cases of osteoarthritis affecting the knees or hands. If further pain relief is required, an oral NSAID, selective inhibitor of COX-2 or opioid should be considered; a proton pump inhibitor should be taken with an NSAID or selective COX-2 inhibitor to limit the gastrointestinal side-effects. Non-pharmacological measures such as weight-reduction and exercise should be discussed with the patient and actively encouraged to reduce further damage of the affected area.

3 **Disease-modifying antirheumatic drugs (DMARDs) have an immediate therapeutic response**

These agents help slow the progression of rheumatic disease but full therapeutic response can be slow and may not be evident until treatment has been ongoing for between 2 and 6 months. Since rheumatoid arthritis is often unpredictable in the first few months, treatment usually begins with an NSAID (although these only control symptoms) with a DMARD only being introduced once diagnosis, progression, and severity of the condition have been confirmed.

4 **Skeletal muscle relaxants should be prescribed to treat spasm associated with minor injuries**

Skeletal muscle relaxants should be used for the relief of chronic muscle spasm and spasticity associated with chronic illnesses such as multiple sclerosis and should not be prescribed for spasm associated with minor injuries. Many (but not all) of these drugs, such as baclofen and diazepam, act principally on the central nervous system, although some, such as dantrolene, act on peripheral regions. Cannabis extract has both central and peripheral effects. Skeletal muscle relaxants act differently to the muscle relaxants used in anaesthesia, which act by blocking neuromuscular transmission. Skeletal muscle relaxants are effective in most forms of spasticity, although many can cause drowsiness and sedative effects.

5 | **Anticholinesterases reduce neuromuscular transmission in myasthenia gravis**

Anticholinesterase drugs enhance neuromuscular transmission in the autoimmune disorder myasthenia gravis. They prolong the action of the neurotransmitter acetylcholine by inhibiting the acetylcholinesterase enzyme (which usually degrades acetylcholine). Overdosing of these drugs can cause excessive stimulation of the acetylcholine receptors by acetylcholine and impair neuromuscular transmission; this may result in a cholinergic crisis, which presents as muscle weakness. Other adverse effects include abdominal cramps, nausea, diarrhoea and vomiting, and are due to stimulation of muscarinic receptors, although these can be counteracted by administering atropine.

MULTIPLE CHOICE

Correct answers identified in bold italics.

6 | **Which of the following does not describe a mechanism of action for antigout drugs?**

a) drugs that act on the joint
b) *drugs that act on the GI system*
c) drugs that reduce uric acid synthesis
d) drugs that increase the excretion of uric acid by the kidneys

Gout is a metabolic disorder caused by an accumulation of uric acid in the blood. Uric acid is normally excreted in the urine but if the body produces too much uric acid or it is not effectively excreted in the urine, it builds up, forming very small crystals in and around the joints. Treatment aims to relieve symptoms of pain and prevent recurrent attacks in the future by reducing concentrations of uric acid in the blood. Drugs that act on the joint aim to reduce inflammation and include NSAIDs, which may be used as short-term treatments for acute gout. Colchicine is also effective in relieving pain associated with acute gout by reducing the accumulation of neutrophils at the affected joint. Drugs such as allopurinol are effective in reducing synthesis of uric acid by inhibiting the enzyme responsible for its synthesis. Patients with renal impairment can use allopurinol, since it does not rely on the kidneys to exert its effects. Other drugs increase the renal excretion of uric acid by decreasing its reabsorption back into the blood at the kidneys. This is the mechanism of action of sulfinpyrazone, which may be used instead of allopurinol or in addition to it.

7 **Local corticosteroid injection is not recommended as a treatment for:**

a) rheumatoid arthritis   b) tennis elbow

c) carpal tunnel syndrome   *d) inflammation of the Achilles tendon*

Injection of corticosteroid at the site of inflammation in joints (such as rheumatoid arthritis), soft tissue disorders (such as tennis elbow), and nerve entrapment conditions (such as carpal tunnel syndrome) can relieve pain and increase mobility at the site. The treatment of tendinitis (inflamed tendons) with local corticosteroid involves injection into the sheath surrounding the tendon rather than into the tendon itself. It is not recommended as a treatment for inflammation of the Achilles tendon due to the absence of a true sheath around the tendon and injection at this site may lead to rupture of the Achilles tendon. Common corticosteroids used for local injection include dexamethasone, hydrocortisone, beta-methasone, prednisolone, and methylprednisolone.

8 **Which of the following compounds may be used in second-line anti-arthritic treatments?**

a) gold b) silver c) mercury d) carbon dioxide

Compounds containing gold are considered second-line treatment for arthritis. Second-line treatments (including gold, antimalarials, and penicillamine) are slower acting and potentially more toxic than the NSAIDs. Therefore, all second-line options are only recommended when treatment with NSAIDs has been unsuccessful. When used to treat rheumatoid arthritis, gold is given as sodium aurothiomalate via intramuscular injection. A number of patients report adverse effects such as skin rash and pruritus when undergoing gold therapy; in these circumstances, treatment should be discontinued. Penicillamine has a similar action to gold and although side-effects are common, fewer patients are forced to discontinue treatment due to such issues.

9 **Cannabis extract is licensed as a treatment for which musculoskeletal disorder?**

a) spinal cord injuries   b) nocturnal cramp

c) multiple sclerosis   d) osteomyelitis

Cannabis extract is licensed as a skeletal muscle relaxant for moderate-to-severe multiple sclerosis in patients who have not responded to other forms of skeletal muscle relaxants. If an adequate response is not achieved within four weeks of treatment, it should be discontinued. It has many side-effects, including (but not limited to) modified appetite (increase or decrease), nausea, vomiting, diarrhoea, constipation, taste disturbances, mood disturbances, amnesia, depression, dry mouth, and mouth ulcers. Treatment with cannabis extract is contra-indicated in patients with a family history of psychiatric disorders.

10 **Which of the following is considered first-line treatment for pain associated with osteoarthritis and soft tissues disorders?**

a) NSAIDs
b) mild opioids
c) moderate opioids
d) *paracetamol*

For relief of pain associated with osteoarthritis and soft tissues disorders, paracetamol is usually the preferred treatment. It may be combined with a topical NSAID when treating pain in the hand or knee. If paracetamol fails to have an adequate therapeutic effect, an oral NSAID should be administered, which can be taken instead of paracetamol or in combination with it. If an oral NSAID does not provide adequate pain relief, an opioid analgesic may be prescribed but patients should be advised of the potential adverse side-effects with opioids (see Figure 2.1 – The Three-Step Analgesic Ladder). For patients with GI disturbances where an NSAID may be contra-indicated, an opioid analgesic may be considered before an NSAID.

FILL IN THE BLANKS

11 ***Azothioprine*** **is an immunosuppressant that may be used to treat severe, progressive rheumatoid arthritis.**

Azothioprine is a second-line anti-arthritic treatment that should only be used to treat severe, progressive rheumatoid arthritis when the patient has not responded to other treatments. It should be administered in combination with NSAIDs but other second-line treatments such as anti-malarial, gold, and penicillamine should be discontinued. Patients should have a regular blood count to monitor for thrombocytopenia and neutropenia. Adverse effects include nausea, vomiting, and diarrhoea, which usually occur early in treatment and may lead to withdrawal of treatment.

12 **The enzyme** ***hyaluronidase*** **can be used to make tissues more permeable to injected fluids.**

Hyaluronidase increases the permeability of connective tissue to fluids by catalysing the breakdown of hyaluronic acid in the body. It may be used to enhance the absorption and dispersion of subcutaneous or intramuscular injections, subcutaneous infusions or local anaesthetics. It may also be used to enhance the resorption of blood or excess fluids. Hyaluronidase should not be injected into or around an infected or acutely inflamed area, as this increases the risk of spreading a localized infection.

13 ***Cyclosporin*** **may be classified as a disease-modifying antirheumatic drug (DMARD).**

Cyclosporin is a potent immunosuppressant drug that is considered a disease-modifying antirheumatic drug (DMARD) because it not only decreases the pain and swelling of arthritis but may also limit joint damage, thereby slowing disease progression. DMARDs differ from NSAIDs, since NSAIDs only provide symptomatic relief of joint pain by reducing inflammation. Patients with suspected inflammatory joint disease should initially be treated with NSAIDs until diagnosis is confirmed. Upon positive diagnosis of inflammatory joint disease, treatment with DMARDs should commence immediately to reduce joint damage and control symptoms. Other DMARDs include methotrexate, azathioprine, and cyclophosphamide.

14 **Pyridostigmine bromide is used in the treatment of _myasthenia gravis_.**

Pyridostigmine bromide is an anticholinesterase that prevents the breakdown of acetylcholine (which is involved in muscle contraction). Pyridostigmine bromide is used to treat certain muscle conditions such as when the muscles are weak. Myasthenia gravis is an autoimmune disease characterized by weak muscles that tire easily. Pyridostigmine bromide works by delaying the breakdown of acetylcholine when it is released from nerve endings, meaning more is available for the muscle receptors, which improves muscle strength. Common side-effects of this medication include nausea, vomiting, diarrhoea, abdominal cramps, and increased production of saliva. Other anticholinesterase drugs used in the treatment of myasthenia gravis include neostigmine and distigmine. Neostigmine is stronger and has a quicker onset of action than pyridostigmine bromide but it has a shorter duration of action – because of its smoother action, pyridostigmine bromide is preferred to neostigmine. Distigmine has the longest action but an increased risk of cholinergic crisis due to the accumulation of the drug.

15 **Diclofenac is an _NSAID_ drug used to treat pain and inflammation associated with rheumatic disorders.**

Diclofenac is classified as a selective COX-2 inhibitor and has a similar action and side-effects to naproxen. As a selective COX-2 inhibitor it has a better GI tolerance, although it does carry an increased risk of thrombotic events such as myocardial infarction or cerebrovascular accident. Diclofenac and ibuprofen are the recommended NSAIDs for the treatment of mild-to-moderate dental (and other orofacial) pain and inflammatory conditions.

MATCH THE TERMS

16 Prednisolone	**B.** corticosteroid
17 Diclofenac	**E.** NSAID
18 Diazepam	**F.** skeletal muscle relaxant
19 Cyclosporin	**A.** DMARD (immune response modulator)
20 Allopurinol	**D.** uric acid lowering agent
21 Pyridostigmine bromide	**C.** anticholinesterase (enhances neuromuscular transmission)

Figure 4.1 Drugs used in the treatment of musculoskeletal disorders

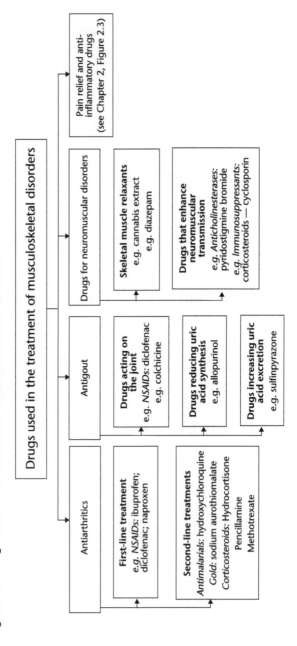

5 Drugs and the nervous system and special senses

INTRODUCTION

The nervous system is the primary mode of rapid communication between the organs and systems of the body. It consists of the brain, spinal cord (the central nervous system), and the peripheral nerves.

Neurological disorders, such as epilepsy and dementias (Alzheimer's disease, Parkinson's disease), are usually caused by structural, biochemical or electrical abnormalities of the nervous system and can result in a range of symptoms. They are usually treated with drugs that alter the neuronal activity in the brain to control symptoms. Mental health disorders are often due to a chemical imbalance of neurotransmitters in the brain. Drugs can be used to change the balance of these chemicals in the brain but can also have an effect on the patient's emotions.

Since many patients seek medical attention for the control and eradication of pain, it is important for nurses to understand the mechanisms by which pain medication exerts an analgesic effect. This is also important for understanding the potential side-effects and drug interactions that can occur. There are two types of pain that the body may experience: nociceptive pain and neuropathic pain. Most analgesic pain medications block the nociceptive signal to the brain. Neuropathic pain is caused by a disorder of the nervous system (it does not involve nociceptors); since the nervous system is actually causing the pain, it can make pain more difficult to identify and treat. Pain is often classified as acute or chronic, which also impacts on its pharmacological management and treatment.

Useful resources

Nurses! Test Yourself in Pathophysiology
Chapter 5

Nurses! Test Yourself in Anatomy and Physiology
Chapter 5

Essentials of Pharmacology for Nurses, 2nd edition
Chapters 3, 7 and 8

TRUE OR FALSE?

Are the following statements true or false?

1 | Non-pharmacological treatment is usually discouraged when treating mental health disorders.

2 | Opioid drugs utilize the body's natural analgesic system to provide pain relief.

3 | The effects of sympathomimetic drugs are similar to those produced by the parasympathetic nervous system.

4 | Beta-adrenergic blockers specifically block the action of adrenaline on beta-adrenergic receptors.

5 | Antipsychotic drugs produce side-effects similar to those of Parkinson's disease.

6 | Nitrazepam is an anxiolytic drug.

7 | An epidural route is an effective method for providing local anaesthesia.

8 | Neuropathic pain can be successfully treated with conventional analgesia.

MULTIPLE CHOICE

Identify one correct answer for each of the following.

9 Most drugs used in treating mental health disorders target:

a) myelin sheaths of neurones

b) dendrites of neurones

c) synapses between neurones

d) the cell body within neurones

10 Which of the following actions is not triggered by a beta-blocker drug?

a) increase in blood pressure

b) bronchoconstriction

c) slow heart rate and reduced cardiac output

d) alleviate symptoms of anxiety

11 Involuntary muscle spasm may be relieved using which type of drug?

a) adenosine

b) adrenaline

c) anticholinesterases

d) antimuscarinics

12 Which of the following is not a symptom associated with opioid drugs?

a) decrease in GI motility

b) nausea and vomiting

c) respiratory depression

d) psychological depression

13 The main drug used in the prophylaxis and treatment of mania is:

a) carbamazepine

b) diazepam

c) lithium

d) nitrazepam

14 Which of the following types of drugs is not an antidepressant?

a) monoamine oxidase inhibitors

b) anxiolytics

c) selective serotonin reuptake inhibitors

d) tricyclic antidepressants

FILL IN THE BLANKS

Fill in the blanks in each statement using the options in the box below.
Not all of them are required, so choose carefully!

adrenaline	anticholinesterase
antidiuretic	potassium
anti-epileptic	sympathomimetics
antidepressant	noradrenaline
sodium	local
general	antipsychotic

15 The main target for local anaesthetics is the _____ channels of nociceptor neurones.

16 _____ drugs have a sedative and tranquilizing effect on the mind.

17 Alpha-adrenergic receptor blockers prevent the vasoconstriction triggered by _____.

18 The effects of acetylcholine can be prolonged and intensified using an _____ drug.

19 _____ medicines target the imbalance of excitatory and inhibitory electrical stimulation by neurones in the brain.

20 A _____ anaesthetic provides pain relief by blocking all nerve signals to the brain.

MATCH THE TERMS

Match each of the following drugs with the listed pharmacological/clinical functions:

A. tricyclic antidepressant

B. hypnotic

C. selective serotonin reuptake inhibitor

D. non-opioid analgesic

E. second-generation antipsychotic

F. anxiolytic (benzodiazapine)

G. monoamine oxidase inhibitor

H. antimanic

I. GABA inhibitor

J. mild opioid analgesic

K. calcium channel blocker

L. sodium channel blocker

| 21 | Zopiclone | | 27 | Amitriptyline |

| 22 | Olanzapine | | 28 | Phenytoin |

| 23 | Fentanyl | | 29 | Aspirin |

| 24 | Ethosuximide | | 30 | Fluoxetine |

| 25 | Valproate | | 31 | Vigabatrin |

| 26 | Diazepam | | 32 | Citalopram |

ANSWERS

TRUE OR FALSE?

1 **Non-pharmacological treatment is usually discouraged when treating mental health disorders**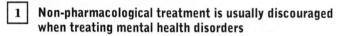

A lot of mental health drugs produce many side-effects and can cause dependence. Thus the prescription of these drugs is advised with caution, especially when a non-pharmacological alternative is available, as this can reduce the side-effects and possibility of developing either biochemical dependence (associated with the limbic system in the brain which regulates emotions) or psychological dependence. When prescribed, it is advised that doses of mental health drugs should be as low as possible and for as short a time as possible.

2 **Opioid drugs utilize the body's natural analgesic system to provide pain relief**

The body's natural analgesic mechanism is not well understood but it is believed to release opioid-like peptides that block the transmission of pain signals at the synapses of nociceptor neurones (coming from the pain receptor) in the spinal cord, thus suppressing the pain sensation. Opioid analgesic drugs such as codeine and morphine are similar in molecular structure to the natural opioid-like peptides (such as endorphins or enkephalins) and therefore can utilize this mechanism to suppress the experience of pain. Opioid analgesics are the strongest and most effective painkillers currently available.

3 **The effects of sympathomimetic drugs are similar to those produced by the parasympathetic nervous system**

Sympathomimetic drugs (also known as adrenoceptor agonists) have effects similar to those produced by the substances liberated by the sympathetic nervous system – adrenaline and noradrenaline. The family includes selective beta$_2$ agonists and other adrenoceptor agonists, namely adrenaline (or ephedrine) and noradrenaline. When adrenaline is administered (as a drug), it acts on the sympathetic receptors of the visceral organs in a similar way to that of the natural neurotransmitter adrenaline. As a drug, adrenaline is degraded by stomach acid and thus it is not suitable for oral administration. It is usually administered by subcutaneous or intramuscular injection (action is more rapid following IM injection). Adrenaline increases the force and rate of the heart, increases systolic blood pressure, relaxes smooth muscle, and increases blood glucose. Noradrenaline produces widespread vasoconstriction, increasing both systolic and diastolic blood pressure. Beta agonists stimulate the beta receptors in the same manner as adrenaline and noradrenaline. Beta$_2$ agonist drugs predominantly stimulate the beta$_2$-adrenergic receptors; therefore they are most effective in the respiratory system but can have a minor effect on the heart.

4 | **Beta-adrenergic blockers specifically block the action of adrenaline on beta-adrenergic receptors**

Beta-adrenergic receptor blockers (beta-blockers) block the action of both neurotransmitters of the sympathetic nervous system: adrenaline and noradrenaline. Some beta-blockers predominantly target beta$_1$ receptors found in heart tissue, and are called selective (or cardioselective) beta-blockers. Other beta-blockers are non-selective because they block both beta$_1$ and beta$_2$ receptors; these drugs affect cells in the heart, the bronchi, and the peripheral blood vessels (since beta$_2$ receptors are located in the bronchi and peripheral vessels). Beta-blockers differ according to their speed of onset, duration of action, and their site of elimination.

5 | **Antipsychotic drugs produce side-effects similar to those of Parkinson's disease**

Antipsychotic drugs (also known as neuroleptics) are dopamine antagonists, meaning they block dopamine receptors in the substantia nigra in the brain, which limits the effects of the neurotransmitter dopamine. Blocking the action of dopamine causes symptoms such as involuntary movement, tremors, and lack of motor coordination; these are also symptoms of Parkinson's disease, which is characterized by a degeneration of dopamine production by the substantia nigra. Antipsychotic drugs also bind to the receptors of other neurotransmitters, including serotonin (5-HT), acetylcholine, and adrenaline, causing a range of side-effects including headache, confusion, drowsiness, dizziness, and hypotension.

6 | **Nitrazepam is an anxiolytic drug**

Nitrazepam is a hypnotic (sleep inducing) agent commonly used to treat insomnia. It belongs to the benzodiazepine family of drugs, which also includes flurazepam and temazepam. Zopiclone is a non-benzodiazepine hypnotic that has very similar activity and side-effects but a different chemical structure. If the insomnia is due to anxiety, it is common to prescribe diazepam, which is an anxiolytic hypnotic drug. Nitrazepam and flurazepam have a longer duration of action than temazepam, meaning patients should be careful when driving or operating machinery the morning after use. Hypnotics are only recommended for short-term use.

7 | **An epidural route is an effective method for providing local anaesthesia**

An epidural provides local anaesthesia by injecting the anaesthetic drug into the epidural space surrounding the spinal cord. Epidural analgesia provides strong pain relief to the regions served by nerves in that area of the spinal cord. The areas that can be numbed by an epidural include the chest, abdomen, pelvis, and legs. The extent of the pain relief and numbness depends on the type of and amount of anaesthetic used. Epidurals have been routinely used for many years and are widely accepted as an effective method of pain relief during and after certain types of surgery and during labour. Lidocaine and bupivacaine are commonly used in epidurals for surgical procedures such as hip replacement. Bupivacaine is the preferred epidural analgesia during labour but at lower concentrations than for surgery. There are a number of risks associated with the procedure, including infection and puncture of the dura (surrounding the spinal cord), although both are rare.

8 | **Neuropathic pain can be successfully treated with conventional analgesia**

Neuropathic pain is not generated through stimulation of nociceptor neurones by injury or inflammation, thus neuropathic pain is not signalled through normal neural pain pathways and cannot be treated with common analgesic drugs. Instead, it is triggered by neurological dysfunction, which makes treatment difficult because this pain mechanism is not well understood. Conditions such as shingles, multiple sclerosis, and diabetic neuropathy cause neuropathic pain. Occasionally regular analgesics such as NSAIDs or paracetamol may be successful in treating neuropathic pain but their effects are erratic and unpredictable. Alternatively, certain tricyclic antidepressants (TCAs) or anti-epileptics may be prescribed but the effectiveness of both is variable.

MULTIPLE CHOICE

Correct answers identified in bold italics.

9 | **Most drugs used in treating mental health disorders target:**

a) myelin sheaths of neurones
b) dendrites of neurones
c) *synapses between neurones*
d) the cell body within neurones

The majority of drugs used to treat mental health disorders target the synapses between neurones located in the deep emotional centres of the brain in the limbic system. Drugs act to amplify or suppress the activity of specific neurotransmitters at the synapse. The pharmacological effect depends on the nature of the neurotransmitter, namely whether its natural effects are excitatory or inhibitory. Excitatory neurotransmitters, such as adrenaline and noradrenaline, stimulate the brain. If the neurotransmitter is excitatory, amplifying its activity will produce an increase in excitation at the synapse; if an excitatory neurotransmitter is suppressed, its action is inhibited and the excitatory effect decreases. Inhibitory neurotransmitters, such as serotonin or gamma-aminobutyric acid (GABA), calm the mind and balance mood. If an inhibitory neurotransmitter is amplified, the inhibition effect is increased, while suppressing an inhibitory neurotransmitter will decrease its inhibitory effect.

10 **Which of the following actions is not triggered by a beta-blocker drug?**

a) *increase in blood pressure*

b) bronchoconstriction

c) slow heart rate and reduced cardiac output

d) alleviate symptoms of anxiety

Beta-blockers inhibit the vasoconstriction triggered by the binding of adrenaline to receptors in peripheral blood vessels. The associated relaxation of the smooth muscle lining the blood vessels widens the lumen of the vessels, thus reducing blood pressure. Blocking beta$_1$ receptors in the heart reduces the heart rate, cardiac output, and electrical conduction in heart muscle. Blocking beta$_2$ receptors may cause bronchospasm in asthmatic patients because the smooth muscle of the bronchi constricts in the absence of adrenaline (or a beta$_2$ agonist drug). Although the exact mechanism of action is unknown, beta-blockers (such as propranolol) are often prescribed to alleviate the symptoms of anxiety, since many of such symptoms (namely palpitations, sweating, and tremor) are mediated through the sympathetic nervous system.

11 **Involuntary muscle spasm may be relieved using which type of drug?**

a) adenosine   b) adrenaline

c) anticholinesterases   d) *antimuscarinics*

Antimuscarinic (anticholinergic) drugs relax smooth muscle, relieving spasm. Atropine is an antimuscarinic that inhibits the action of acetylcholine released from parasympathetic nerves, so it relaxes involuntary spasm in smooth muscle. It is useful in the treatment of irritable bowel syndrome, diverticular disease, and renal colic. Atropine is also commonly used to dilate the pupil of the eye for examination. Ipratropium is a derivative of atropine, commonly used in the treatment of bronchospasm to dilate the airways (see Chapter 8).

12 **Which of the following is not a symptom associated with opioid drugs?**

a) decrease in GI motility   b) nausea and vomiting

c) respiratory depression   d) *psychological depression*

The strong effects of opioids on the nervous system is associated with a number of side-effects, such as nausea and vomiting (especially after initial administration), respiratory depression (probably due to the respiratory centre's reduced sensitivity to carbon dioxide, which stimulates breathing), and constipation (particularly associated with codeine). Opioid drugs, especially morphine, tend to produce feelings of euphoria rather than depression, similar to the effects of the illegal drug heroin.

13 **The main drug used in the prophylaxis and treatment of mania is:**

a) carbamazepine   b) diazepam

c) lithium   d) nitrazepam

Mania is characterized as a state of extreme excitement often accompanied by increased energy. It is exhibited by patients with bipolar illness who experience recurrent mood swings of mania and depression (formerly known as manic-depression). Although its mechanism of action is not known, lithium is the main drug used in the prophylaxis and treatment of mania. It is successful in the prophylactic management of bipolar illness, recurrent depression, schizophrenia, and aggressive behaviours. It has a number of common side-effects, including abdominal pain, nausea, thirst, polyuria, impaired urinary concentration, weight gain, oedema, fine tremor, and a metallic taste in the mouth (which usually subsides). Its use requires regular monitoring to avoid toxicities associated with the thyroid gland and kidneys. Carbamazepine is a sodium-channel blocker associated with the treatment of epilepsy. Diazepam is an anxiolytic used in the treatment of anxiety. Nitrazepam is a hypnotic used to treat insomnia.

14 **Which of the following types of drugs is not an antidepressant?**

a) monoamine oxidase inhibitors

b) anxiolytics

c) selective serotonin reuptake inhibitors

d) tricyclic antidepressants

Anxiolytics are used to treat unnatural anxieties caused by a series of physiological and psychological events of the sympathetic nervous system in response to a stressful situation. There are three main groups of antidepressant drugs: (1) monoamine oxidase inhibitors (MAOIs), (2) selective serotonin reuptake inhibitors (SSRIs), and (3) tricyclic antidepressants (TCAs). They all act on neurones in the brain that release the neurotransmitters serotonin (5-HT) and noradrenaline, increasing the amount of these neurotransmitters available at the synapses. Since these neurotransmitters are associated with mood, increasing their availability at the synapses can relieve depression associated with reduced levels. TCAs and SSRIs block the reuptake of serotonin and noradrenaline at the synapse, although SSRIs are most specific to serotonin, while MAOIs inhibit the enzyme monoamine oxidase that breaks down dopamine, noradrenaline, and serotonin. MAOIs are used less frequently nowadays due to their side-effects and interactions (with drugs and certain foods).

FILL IN THE BLANKS

15 The main target for local anaesthetics is the _sodium_ channels of nociceptor neurones.

Local anaesthetics block the sodium ion channels found on the membranes of nociceptor neurones. When these channels are blocked, the nerve impulse cannot be transmitted along the axon of the neurone, so the pain signal does not reach the brain and thus the pain sensation is not experienced. Local anaesthetics tend to work on small sensory nociceptor neurones between the pain receptor and the spinal cord rather than major motor neurones, which allows for suppression of pain sensation with only minimal loss of motor function. Commonly used local anaesthetics include lidocaine, bupivacaine, and tetracaine.

16 _Antipsychotic_ drugs have a sedative and tranquilizing effect on the mind.

Antipsychotic drugs are usually only used for serious mental health disorders such as schizophrenia, severe anxiety or unpredictable or violent behaviour; they have a tranquilizing and sedating effect on the mind and are therefore considered to be mood stabilizers. They are classified into the older, first-generation or 'typical' antipsychotics and the newer, second-generation 'atypical' antipsychotics. The first-generation (typical) drugs belong to the phenothiazine group, which are dopamine antagonists that block the dopamine receptors and ultimately stabilize the mood, although their mechanism of action is not well understood. The second-generation (atypical) antipsychotics include risperidone and clozapine and act on a range of receptors including dopamine but have less motor-related side-effects than the first-generation antipsychotic drugs.

17 Alpha-adrenergic receptor blockers prevent the vasoconstriction triggered by _noradrenaline_.

By blocking the alpha-adrenergic receptors, noradrenaline cannot bind to the receptors, thus preventing vasoconstriction. This explains the use of alpha-adrenergic blockers in the treatment of hypertension, since they facilitate the dilation of arterioles and hence reduce blood pressure.

18 The effects of acetylcholine can be prolonged and intensified using an _anticholinesterase_ drug.

Anticholinesterase drugs prolong and intensify the action of the natural parasympathetic neurotransmitter acetylcholine by inhibiting the action of the enzyme acetylcholinesterase, which degrades acetylcholine once it is released from the cholinergic receptor. Anticholinesterase drugs, such as donepezil or rivastigmine are used in the treatment of mild to moderate Alzheimer's Disease.

19 *Anti-epileptic* **medicines target the imbalance of excitatory and inhibitory electrical stimulation by neurones in the brain.**

Epileptic seizures arise when certain nerves in the thalamus and cerebral cortex regions of the brain fire random electrical signals uncontrollably. Symptoms of seizures range from minor lapses in attention to severe muscle spasms and unconsciousness. Anti-epileptic medicines prevent the seizures associated with epilepsy by delaying transmission of nerve impulses in a number of different ways. Some drugs, such as phenytoin, block the sodium ion channels in neurones that are highly excited; others, namely ethosuximide, target calcium ion channels in the relay neurones between the thalamus and cerebral cortex. Other drugs, such as valproate, enhance the inhibitory effects of the GABA neurotransmitter. Many side-effects are associated with anti-epileptic medicines, including nausea, vomiting, confusion, and dizziness. There is a strong association of drug tolerance with certain anti-epileptics, so the initial dose prescribed should be low and only increased to a level sufficient to control seizures. Most anti-epileptic drugs are contra-indicated during pregnancy, as they are associated with certain birth defects.

20 **A** *general* **anaesthetic provides pain relief by blocking all nerve signals to the brain.**

General anaesthesia may be used for pain relief during surgical procedures because it causes complete loss of sensation. The patient is unconscious so that surgery may be performed without pain or distress. A general anaesthetic is essential for some surgical procedures where it may be safer or more comfortable for the patient to be unconscious, usually long operations, or those that could be very painful. A general anaesthetic prevents the brain from recognizing any nerve signals. It may be administered in two ways: (1) by IV injection through a cannula or (2) a gas that is inhaled through a mask. Side-effects are usually short-lived and include nausea or vomiting after surgery, shivering, confusion, memory loss, dizziness, bruising or soreness at the site of injection. On rare occasions patients can develop anaphylaxis due to a general anaesthetic, which must be treated as a medical emergency. General anaesthesia is now commonly used in combination with a sedative to reduce anxiety during induction of the anaesthetic before surgery.

MATCH THE TERMS

21 Zopiclone   **B.** hypnotic

22 Olanzapine   **E.** second-generation antipsychotic

23 Fentanyl   **J.** mild opioid analgesic

24 Ethosuximide   **K.** calcium channel blocker

25 Valproate   **H.** antimanic

26 Diazepam   **F.** anxiolytic (benzodiazapine)

27 Amitriptyline   **A.** tricyclic antidepressant

28 Phenytoin   **L.** sodium channel blocker

29 Aspirin   **D.** non-opioid analgesic

30 Fluoxetine   **G.** monoamine oxidase inhibitor

31 Vigabatrin   **I.** GABA inhibitor

32 Citalopram   **C.** selective serotonin reuptake inhibitor

Figure 5.1 Drugs used in the treatment of nervous system disorders

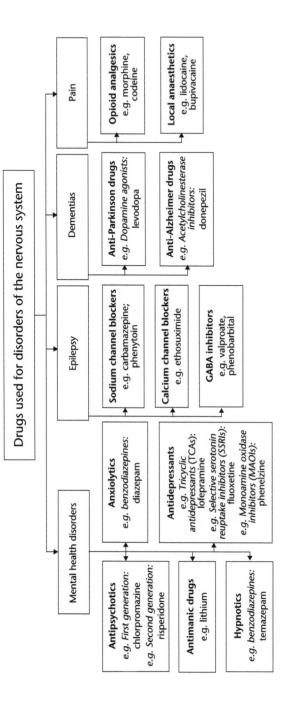

6 Drugs and the endocrine system

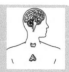

INTRODUCTION

The endocrine system is responsible for chemical coordination and control of communication in the body. It produces and regulates hormones that pass into the bloodstream to be transported to the various tissues of the body where they exert their action, altering the function or activity of the target cells and organs. The pituitary gland is one of the major organs of the system, thus disorders affecting its function can have a major impact of the function of glands targeted by hormones from the pituitary gland. This can subsequently disrupt the physiology of many organs and systems, which can have a widespread impact on normal homeostasis in the body.

Since glands and hormones control a wide range of physiological processes, the associated pathophysiology of disorders and diseases is dissimilar. Therefore, the pharmacology of drugs used to treat disorders of the endocrine system is quite varied. For example, treatment of altered blood glucose concentrations differs considerably from treatment for impaired thyroid function.

Nurses need to recognize and understand the pharmacology of the various drugs associated with treating disorders of the endocrine system, particularly since small amounts of hormones (or their analogues) can have profound effects on the body. In contrast, even minor deficiencies may produce equally profound physiological changes that must be recognized clinically. Nurses must also be able to teach patients about their medication, such as safe and effective administration, potential side-effects, and signs of overdose to be aware of.

Useful resources

Nurses! Test Yourself in Anatomy and Physiology
Chapter 6

Nurses! Test Yourself in Pathophysiology
Chapter 6

Medication for endocrine-related disturbances
http://www.patient.co.uk/leaflets/endocrine_disorder_drugs.htm

TRUE OR FALSE?

Are the following statements true or false?

1 Levothyroxine is typically used to treat hyperthyroidism.

2 Hyperthyroidism is treated by inhibiting the release of thyroid hormones from the thyroid gland.

3 Insulin is inactivated by enzymes in the gastrointestinal tract.

4 The usual treatment for type 2 diabetes is with subcutaneous injection of insulin.

5 Rotation of the injection site is important when administering insulin.

6 Increasing concentrations of circulating progesterone can help to prevent osteoporosis in post-menopausal women.

7 Combined oral contraceptive pills contain synthetic analogues of the natural hormones oestrogen and progesterone.

8 The best time of day to take glucocorticoid drugs is in the evening.

9 Long-term use of topical corticosteroids is not recommended.

10 After treating a patient for 3 weeks or more with an oral steroid drug, withdrawal of the drug must be gradual.

MULTIPLE CHOICE

Identify one correct answer for each of the following.

11 Which of the following is not a mode of action of the combined oral contraceptive pill?

a) inhibits ovulation

b) thickens cervical mucus

c) thins the lining of the uterus

d) inhibits menstruation

12 Which of the following oral hypoglycaemic drugs acts by increasing the amount of insulin produced by the pancreas?

a) biguanides (such as metformin)

b) sulphonylureas (such as gliclazide)

c) thiazolidinediones (such as pioglitazone)

d) dipeptidylpeptidase-4 inhibitors (such as sitagliptin)

13 Which of the following insulin therapies produces a rapid onset of action and a long-lasting effect?

a) biphasic insulins (such as biphasic insulin aspart)

b) short-acting insulins (such as insulin aspart)

c) intermediate-acting insulins (such as isophane insulin)

d) long-acting insulins (such as insulin zinc suspension)

14 Which of the following treatments restores female hormones to pre-menopausal levels?

a) combined oral contraceptive pill

b) progesterone-only pill

c) hormone replacement therapy

d) bisphosphonates

15 Which of the following bone cells are the ultimate target for bisphosphonate drugs?

a) osteoblasts

b) osteoclasts

c) osteocytes

d) all of the above

16 Which of the following is not one of the main glucocorticoid drugs?

a) dexamethasone

b) fludrocortisone

c) hydrocortisone

d) prednisolone

FILL IN THE BLANKS

Fill in the blanks in each statement using the options in the box below.
Not all of them are required, so choose carefully!

hyperglycaemia	progesterone
parathyroid	metformin
hypoglycaemia	thyroid
oestrogen	gliclazide

17 _____ may be prescribed to overweight patients for the treatment of type 2 diabetes.

18 Acute _____ can be treated by administration of oral glucose.

19 A reduction in _____ concentrations is the main cause of osteoporosis in post-menopausal females.

20 _____ hormone is licensed for use as a treatment for osteoporosis.

MATCH THE TERMS

Match each of the drugs with the listed pharmacological/clinical functions:

A. glucocorticoid (steroid)

B. antithyroidhypoglycaemia

C. sulphonylurea (antidiabetic drug)

D. bisphosphonate (antidiabetic drug)

E. thyroid hormone

F. biguanide (antidiabetic drug)

G. intermediate-acting insulin

H. short-acting insulin

---

21 Alendronic acid

22 Prednisolone

23 Isophane insulin

24 Gliclazide

25 Carbimazole

26 Insulin aspart

27 Levothyroxine

28 Metformin

ANSWERS

TRUE OR FALSE?

1 | **Levothyroxine is typically used to treat hyperthyroidism**

Levothyroxine is used to treat hypothyroidism (underactive thyroid) and certain forms of goitre. It is a synthetic form of the natural hormone thyroxine (T4) normally produced by the thyroid gland. When the thyroid gland is not producing enough natural thyroxine, levothyroxine relieves the symptoms associated with thyroxine deficiency, since it increases serum thyroxine concentrations and mimics the action of thyroxine in the body. Common side-effects of levothyroxine include nausea, vomiting, diarrhoea, dizziness, and palpitations. Patients should also be aware of the symptoms associated with an overdose of levothyroxine, which are similar to the symptoms of hyperthyroidism (namely restlessness, flushing, sweating, insomnia, and weight loss) and report these to their doctor.

2 | **Hyperthyroidism is treated by inhibiting the release of thyroid hormones by the thyroid gland**

The thyroid gland releases two hormones, triiodothryonine (T3) and thyroxine (T4), known as the thyroid hormones. Together they regulate the body's metabolic rate. When they are secreted in excessive quantities, the body exhibits a range of symptoms including unexplained weight loss despite an increased appetite, elevated body temperature, protruding eyeballs (exophthalmia), and nervousness. When secretion of the thyroid hormones is inhibited, these symptoms will disappear within 4–8 weeks. The antithyroid drugs used to inhibit thyroid hormones include carbimazole and propylthiouracil, although carbimazole is the preferred option and propylthiouracil should only be used in patients who are intolerant to carbimazole. Iodine (or Lugol's solution) may be used prior to thyroidectomy or in the treatment of thyrotoxicosis (severe hyperthyroidism). It should not be used as a long-term treatment for thyrotoxicosis as its antithyroid activity decreases over time.

3 | **Insulin is inactivated by enzymes in the gastrointestinal tract**

Insulin (both natural and synthetic variants) is a protein-based hormone that can be broken down by enzymes in the GI tract. This is why insulin is administered by injection; the most common route is subcutaneously – usually into the upper thigh, arms, buttocks or abdomen. Insulin is used when diabetic patients have a high blood glucose (hyperglycaemia) to reduce blood glucose concentration. Synthetic insulin mimics the action of natural insulin normally produced by the beta cells of the pancreas. As insulin is a protein it should be stored at 4°C until opened but may be brought to ambient room temperature before use, as the injection of cold insulin is uncomfortable.

4 | The usual treatment for type 2 diabetes is with subcutaneous injection of insulin

The normal treatment for type 1 diabetes is subcutaneous injection of insulin that supplements the body with synthetic insulin, which enables it to maintain normal blood glucose concentrations in the absence of natural insulin that is not being produced by the pancreas. Treating type 2 diabetes is slightly more complex and varies with the severity of the condition. Most patients with type 2 diabetes may be treated with oral antidiabetic drugs, which work in a variety of ways. Some stimulate any residual insulin to be secreted by the pancreas, while others act on muscle and adipose tissue, stimulating it to use glucose from the bloodstream, thereby reducing blood glucose concentrations. Type 2 diabetics are also encouraged to control their condition by dietary adjustments and increasing exercise. In more severe cases of type 2 diabetes that are not well controlled, patients may be required to inject insulin.

5 | Rotation of the injection site is important when administering insulin

Insulin may be administered subcutaneously at a number of sites. It is advisable to rotate the site of injection to reduce the risk of scarring and lipohypertrophy (accumulation of subcutaneous fat tissue), which can interfere with absorption of the drug. The common sites used for insulin injection include the abdominal wall, thigh, and upper lateral gluteal region. The abdominal wall is preferable for short-acting insulin due to its rapid rate of absorption. The thigh is preferable for intermediate-acting formulations due to its slower absorption rate; the upper lateral gluteal region may be used as an alternative to the thigh, which should be avoided when physical activity is planned because the increased blood flow can increase the rate of absorption. The arm is no longer recommended for self-injection due to the risk of injecting into muscle. The site should not be massaged after injection, as this will affect the absorption rate. Nurses are usually responsible for educating patients on how to inject themselves with insulin and it is important to make patients aware that the site of injection should be rotated each time and that the site chosen will influence the rate of insulin absorption into the bloodstream.

6 | Increasing concentrations of circulating progesterone can help to prevent osteoporosis in post-menopausal women

The hormone oestrogen is effective in maintaining bone density, thus supplementing oestrogen concentrations in post-menopausal women can help to prevent osteoporosis. This can be achieved with hormone replacement therapy (HRT), although HRT is not recommended as a first-line therapy for osteoporosis; its use is usually restricted to cases where other treatments are contra-indicated or where there is little response with other treatments.

7 **Combined oral contraceptive pills contain synthetic analogues of the natural hormones oestrogen and progesterone**

The combined oral contraceptive pill (COCP or 'pill') contains synthetic (artificial) versions of the female hormones oestrogen and progesterone, which are naturally produced by the ovaries in pre-menopausal women. It is usually taken as a contraceptive to prevent pregnancy, but can also be used to treat painful or heavy periods, premenstrual syndrome, and endometriosis. When taken as directed, hormonal contraception in the form of the COCP is considered one of the most effective means of contraception. There are many different types and strengths of COCPs, which differ according to their concentrations of synthetic oestrogens and progesterones (progestogens – the synthetic variant of progesterones) in each.

8 **The best time of day to take glucocorticoid drugs is in the evening**

Evening administration of glucocorticoid (steroid) drugs should be avoided, as it can cause insomnia. The ideal time to take steroid drugs is in the morning and with food. The adrenal glands' production of natural glucocorticoids is at a maximum in the morning, and so administration at this time will result in least suppression of their function.

9 **Long-term use of topical corticosteroids is not recommended**

Corticosteroids (steroids), especially betamethasone, can be used to treat many skin conditions. However, their long-term topical application is not recommended, since they can cause thinning of the skin and can increase the risk of a bacterial or fungal skin infection. When applying topical corticosteroids to the skin, gloves should be worn (when possible) and the hands should be washed thoroughly after application, as corticosteroids are readily absorbed through the skin.

10 **After treating a patient for 3 weeks or more with an oral steroid drug, withdrawal of the drug must be gradual**

When treating a patient for 3 weeks or more with oral corticosteroids, withdrawal must be gradual since adrenal suppression (adrenal insufficiency) may have occurred and withdrawing the drug suddenly could mean the patient's body is unable to cope with physiological stress (because the adrenal glands may have stopped producing the natural hormone cortisol that would normally be secreted in times of stress). This can cause adrenal crisis and have life-threatening consequences. When stopping treatment, it should only be under medical supervision where the drug dose is reduced gradually (over a number of weeks) to allow the adrenal glands time to resume production of the natural steroid hormones, which should prevent severe withdrawal symptoms occurring. Patients on oral steroid treatment for more than 3 weeks, or those prescribed high doses of inhaled corticosteroids, should be issued with a steroid treatment card by the pharmacist dispensing their medication.

MULTIPLE CHOICE

Correct answers identified in bold italics.

11 **Which of the following is not a mode of action of the combined oral contraceptive pill?**

a) inhibits ovulation

b) thickens cervical mucus

c) thins the lining of the uterus

d) *inhibits menstruation*

The COCP works in three ways: (1) it alters the hormonal balance in the body, preventing ovulation; (2) it increases the thickness of cervical mucus, making it difficult for sperm to reach the egg for fertilization to occur; and (3) it thins the uterine lining, making it more difficult for a fertilized egg to attach and implant. Although the COCP is safe for most women to use, it is not recommended for people who have a history of thrombosis, breast cancer or those who are very overweight. It is also not recommended for those who smoke heavily. Common side-effects include nausea, mood changes, breast tenderness, and headaches, although such side-effects often subside after a few months or can be overcome by changing the brand of pill being used.

12 **Which of the following oral hypoglycaemic drugs acts by increasing the amount of insulin produced by the pancreas?**

a) biguanides (such as metformin)

b) *sulphonylureas (such as gliclazide)*

c) thiazolidinediones (such as pioglitazone)

d) dipeptidylpeptidase-4 inhibitors (such as sitagliptin)

Sulphonylureas act by augmenting (enhancing) secretion of insulin by the beta cells of the pancreas. These drugs are only effective when there is some residual function still present in the beta cells. Sulphonylureas may only be administered to patients who are not overweight, as they can cause weight gain. They are not recommended in patients for whom metformin is contra-indicated. The choice of sulphonylurea is determined by the side-effects, duration of action, renal function, and the patient's age. Glibenclamide (a sulphonylurea) is not recommended for older adults due to the risk of hypoglycaemia. Biguanides decrease gluconeogenesis and make cells more responsive to insulin. Thiazolidinediones (or glitazones) make cells more sensitive to insulin so that more glucose is removed from the blood, thus reducing blood glucose concentrations; these may be used in combination with metformin. Dipeptidylpeptidase-4 (DPP-4) inhibitors (or gliptins) increase insulin secretion by preventing the breakdown of a natural hormone that helps the body produce insulin but is rapidly broken down; DPP-4 inhibitors also reduce glucagon secretion.

13 **Which of the following insulin therapies produces a rapid onset of action and a long-lasting effect?**

a) *biphasic insulins (such as biphasic insulin aspart)*

b) short-acting insulins (such as insulin aspart)

c) intermediate-acting insulins (such as isophane insulin)

d) long-acting insulins (such as insulin zinc suspension)

Manufactured insulins can be synthesized so that the rate at which they are absorbed into the bloodstream is variable. This impacts on the onset of action and the duration of the drug's therapeutic effect. The range of insulins available can be categorized according to their onset and duration of action. Biphasic insulins are a mixture of intermediate- and fast-acting insulins that combine a rapid onset of action with prolonged therapeutic effects. Short-acting insulins have a rapid onset of action (usually between 30 and 60 minutes) that peaks 2–4 hours after administration and last for up to 8 hours. Intermediate- and long-acting insulins have an onset of action of 1–2 hours, with intermediate-acting insulins peaking 5–8 hours post-treatment and lasting for 12–18 hours while long-acting insulins peak around 6–12 hours post administration and last for up to 36 hours.

14 **Which of the following treatments restores female hormones to pre-menopausal levels?**

a) combined oral contraceptive pill

b) progesterone-only pill

c) *hormone replacement therapy*

d) bisphosphonates

During and after the menopause, many women report a range of symptoms that are attributable to the reduction in natural concentrations of oestrogen and progesterone. Hormone replacement therapy (HRT) involves supplementing these natural hormones to alleviate symptoms. Many formulations are available that vary in their concentrations of synthetic oestrogens and progestogens. HRT may be administered orally or through a transdermal patch, since oestrogens and progestogens are steroid hormones and thus easily absorbed through the skin. The side-effects of HRT are similar to those experienced during the natural, pre-menopausal hormonal cycle in females (cramps, breast tenderness, bloating), although some patients also report nausea and vomiting. HRT has been linked with an increased risk of certain conditions such as CVA, thrombosis and some cancers, namely breast, ovarian, and endometrial.

15 **Which of the following bone cells are the ultimate target for bisphosphonate drugs?**

a) osteoblasts   *b) osteoclasts*

c) osteocytes   d) all of the above

Osteoblast cells build bone whereas osteoclast cells break down old bone that requires replacement. Osteocytes are embedded in bone and provide nutrients to maintain bone as living tissue; they are thought to control the activity of oestoblasts and osteoclasts. When oestrogen concentrations fall post-menopause, the function of osteoblasts declines, although the osteoclasts are not significantly affected by the decrease in oestrogen. This leads to an imbalance between these cells, with more osteoclasts still available to break down bone and fewer osteoblasts present to rebuild new bone; collectively, this leads to the bone matrix becoming spongy and fragile, which increases the risk of fractures. Bisphosphonates have an affinity for calcium and so are naturally absorbed by the bone matrix, which is rich in calcium. When osteoclasts absorb the bone matrix, they also absorb bisphosphonates, which induces apoptosis (cell suicide) in the osteoclast. This reduces the number of osteoclasts and therefore corrects the imbalance between osteoblasts and osteoclasts and helps to maintain bone density and reduce the likelihood of fractures associated with osteoporosis. Bone density may also be reduced by diseases such as hyperparathyroidism and the long-term use of corticosteroid drugs (used for the treatment of rheumatoid arthritis).

16 **Which of the following is not one of the main glucocorticoid drugs?**

a) dexamethasone   *b) fludrocortisone*

c) hydrocortisone   d) prednisolone

The main glucocorticoid drugs are dexamethasone, hydrocortisone, and prednisolone, each of which may be administered orally, topically or parenterally. Beclometasone is also an important glucocorticoid, although it is administered by inhalation. Fludrocortisone belongs to the family of mineralocorticoid drugs that are mainly used to treat adrenal insufficiency disorders but are often used in conjunction with a glucocorticoid for replacement therapy. Therapeutically, glucocorticoids may be used to suppress certain disease processes such as anti-inflammatory conditions, certain tumours or allergic responses (and immune suppression). Prolonged use of high-strength glucocorticoid drugs has many unwanted side-effects, including oedema, 'moon face', muscle wasting, gastric disturbances, suppression of the immune system and inflammatory response, thinning of the skin and bone, hypertension, reduced stress responses, and growth retardation in children.

FILL IN THE BLANKS

17 *__Metformin__* **may be prescribed to overweight patients for the treatment of type 2 diabetes.**

Metformin is the only biguanide currently available. It is often used as the treatment of choice for type 2 diabetes when a strict diet and exercise regime has failed (although patients are encouraged to maintain a strict diet and exercise regime while taking metformin). It can be taken by overweight patients because, unlike many treatments for this condition, it does not have the associated side-effect of causing weight gain. Known side-effects include nausea and diarrhoea. Metformin acts by enabling cells to increase their use of glucose and inhibiting gluconeogenesis (synthesis of glucose from non-carbohydrate sources such as amino acids or fats), which reduces the amount of glucose released into the blood by the liver. It will only be effective if some residual function remains in the beta cells of the pancreas. Metformin may be prescribed in combination with some of the other oral hypoglycaemic drugs when treatment alone has been unsuccessful.

18 **Acute *__hypoglycaemia__* can be treated by administration of oral glucose.**

Acute hypoglycaemia (low blood glucose concentrations) may occur when a diabetic patient has not eaten for a considerable period of time, has exercised strenuously or has overdosed on insulin or antidiabetic medication. Acute hypoglycaemia is usually treated by administering 10–20 g of oral glucose in liquid (such as fruit juice but not a diet version) or solid form (such as dextrose tablets, sugar or chocolate). Either treatment will rapidly raise the concentration of glucose in the bloodstream and should be followed with a carbohydrate-rich snack or meal to prevent recurrence. If glucose cannot be administered orally because the patient is unconscious, an injection of the hormone glucagon may be administered (subcutaneously, intramuscularly or intravenously), which will quickly raise blood glucose concentrations and restore consciousness. Patients should monitor their blood glucose regularly throughout the day, be educated to recognize the symptoms of hypoglycaemia, and encouraged to carry a supply of liquid or solid glucose at all times to counteract symptoms quickly. Although rare, non-diabetic people may also suffer from acute hypoglycaemia that can be triggered by binge drinking, malnutrition or certain illnesses, such as Addison's disease. In such cases, the immediate treatment is the same; however, the underlying condition will also need to be treated.

19 **A reduction in *__oestrogen__* concentrations is the main cause of osteoporosis in post-menopausal females.**

Bone density is affected by diet, exercise, and hormones. It reaches its peak between the ages of 20–30 years, after which it slowly declines, meaning osteoporosis is usually considered a disease of older adults.

It is more common in older females due to the decline in levels of oestrogen, which helps bone formation, in the body after menopause. The bisphosphonate family of drugs are recommended for osteoporosis, since they are naturally absorbed by the bone matrix.

20 *Parathyroid* **hormone is licensed for use as a treatment for osteoporosis.**

The parathyroid gland (located on the posterior of the thyroid gland) secretes two hormones involved in the regulation of serum calcium concentrations: calcitonin and parathyroid hormone (PTH). Endogenous calcitonin conserves bone by inhibiting the function of osteoclasts. It is available as a synthetic hormone called salcatonin, which can be used in the treatment of osteoporosis but also prophylactically in patients who are immobilized for a prolonged period of time. It may at first seem odd to recommend parathyroid hormone as a treatment for osteoporosis, since it normally removes calcium from bone (which can lead to osteoporosis) and increase serum calcium; however, PTH has recently been licensed as a treatment for post-menopausal osteoporosis, corticosteroid-induced osteoporosis, and osteoporosis in males. Its mechanism of action centres on the daily subcutaneous injection of PTH, which has been found to stimulate the function of osteoblasts (which build bone) and therefore corrects the imbalance with the bone-breaking osteoclasts, which helps increase bond density and therefore reduces the risk of fractures associated with osteoporosis.

 MATCH THE TERMS

21 Alendronic acid   **D.** bisphosphonate (antidiabetic drug)

22 Prednisolone   **A.** glucocorticoid (steroid)

23 Isophane insulin   **G.** intermediate acting insulin

24 Gliclazide   **C.** sulphonylurea (antidiabetic drug)

25 Carbimazole   **B.** antithyroid

26 Insulin aspart   **H.** short-acting insulin

27 Levothyroxine   **E.** thyroid hormone

28 Metformin   **F.** biguanide (antidiabetic drug)

Figure 6.1 Drugs targeting the glands and hormones of the endocrine system

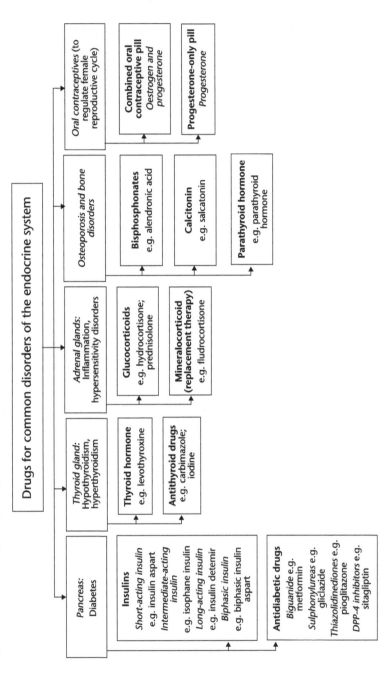

7 Drugs and the cardiovascular system

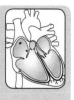

INTRODUCTION

The cardiovascular system is the main circulatory system responsible for transporting blood around the body to the organs and tissues. It consists of the heart, all the blood vessels that supply the organs and tissues with vital oxygen and glucose, and the blood itself. Disease of the cardiovascular system can arise in any part of the system and can sometimes be a symptom of a different underlying condition; for example, hypertension can develop as a complication of renal disease or diabetes.

Coronary heart disease (CHD) is the biggest killer in the UK and often develops as a complication of another chronic condition such as diabetes. There are a number of other major disorders of the cardiovascular system that may require drug treatment, such as cardiac arrhythmias, cardiac failure, cardiac ischaemia, and hypertension. Many of the drugs used in treating cardiac disorders are indicated in more than one type of cardiac disorder (and in disorders of other systems); for example, beta-blockers are used to prevent arrhythmias, alleviate angina, and to treat hypertension and heart failure.

Many patients taking medicines for cardiovascular conditions will remain on medication for the rest of their life, so it is important that they are familiar with their drugs and are aware of what each drug is for. It is important to stress to patients the need to take their medication regularly as prescribed, and that they should report any side-effects or adverse effects they experience.

Useful resources

Nurses! Test Yourself in Essential Calculation Skills
Chapters 1 and 2

Nurses! Test Yourself in Anatomy and Physiology
Chapters 1 and 2

Further Essentials of Pharmacology for Nurses
Chapter 1

TRUE OR FALSE?

Are the following statements true or false?

1 Patients with resistant heart failure may experience a marked decrease in blood pressure when angiotensin-converting enzyme (ACE) inhibitors and diuretics are taken concurrently.

2 Lidocaine can be administered orally to reduce cardiac arrthymias.

3 Cardioselective beta-blockers target the beta$_2$ adrenoceptors in the myocardium.

4 Patients with coronary heart disease may be prescribed anticoagulant drugs.

5 Beta-blockers and calcium channel blockers act as positive inotropes.

6 Alpha-adrenoceptor blockers are generally used in combination with other antihypertensive drugs when treating resistant hypertension.

7 Nitrate drugs act directly on all the involuntary muscles of the body causing them to relax.

8 Methyldopa lowers blood pressure by acting on parasympathetic nervous activity in the brain.

9 Anticoagulant drugs can be used to prevent and treat an arterial or venous thrombosis.

MULTIPLE CHOICE

Identify one correct answer for each of the following.

10 Which of the following types of drugs is not normally used to treat cardiac failure?

a) diuretics

b) ACE inhibitors

c) antiplatelet treatments

d) positive inotropic drugs

11 Verapamil, used to treat hypertension, angina, and certain arrhythmias, is classified as which type of drug?

a) beta-blocker

b) ACE inhibitor

c) cardiac glycoside

d) calcium channel blocker

12 Which of the following types of drugs would not be used to treat cardiac arrhythmias?

a) ACE inhibitors

b) beta-blockers

c) cardiac glycosides

d) calcium channel blockers

13 ACE inhibitor drugs lower blood pressure by targeting which enzyme system?

a) coagulation cascade

b) renin-angiotensin system

c) complement system

d) digestive enzymes

14 Furosemide, which can be used to treat congestive cardiac failure, acts on which part of the kidneys?

a) nephron

b) proximal convoluted tubule

c) loop of Henlé

d) distal convoluted tubule

15 Patients on long-acting or transdermal nitrate formulations can rapidly develop:

a) tolerance

b) toxicity

c) adverse reaction

d) drowsiness

16 In the treatment of shock, noradrenaline primarily acts on which adrenergic receptors?

a) $beta_2$ adrenoceptor

b) $beta_1$ adrenoceptor

c) $alpha_2$ adrenoceptor

d) $alpha_1$ adrenoceptor

17 How do statins work to lower serum cholesterol concentrations?

a) prevent absorption of saturated fats from the diet

b) inhibit an enzyme involved in production of cholesterol by the body

c) prevent storage of excess dietary fats

d) inhibit glucagon secretion

18 Aspirin is classified as an antiplatelet drug. How does it work?

a) stimulates aggregation of platelets

b) inhibits formation of platelets

c) inhibits binding of platelets to fibrin

d) inhibits breakdown of platelets

FILL IN THE BLANKS

Fill in the blanks in each statement using the options in the box below.
Not all of them are required, so choose carefully!

diuretics	haemoglobin
beta-blockers	oxygen
antidiuretics	respiratory
inotropes	sympathomimetics
vasodilators	thrombolytic
diabetes	adenosine

19 _____ are the most important drugs for relieving cardiac failure.

20 _____ – _____ may be prescribed to reduce hypertension.

21 Drugs that increase the lumen of arterioles are called _____.

22 Non-selective beta-blockers are contra-indicated for patients with certain _____ conditions.

23 _____ are used in the treatment of shock to improve tissue perfusion.

24 _____ is usually the treatment of choice for terminating supraventricular tachycardia.

25 In emergencies such as myocardial infarction, _____ agents may be administered to disperse a clot.

26 Iron-deficiency anaemia is characterized by a low_____ concentration.

MATCH THE TERMS

Match each of the drugs with the listed pharmacological/clinical functions:

A. anticoagulant

B. thrombolytic (fibrinolytic)

C. cardioselective beta-blocker

D. antihypertensive (thiazide diuretic)

E. positive inotrope

F. calcium channel blocker

G. lipid regulator

H. antiangina (short-acting)

I. ACE inhibitor

---

27 Fosinopril sodium

28 Reteplase

29 Simvastatin

30 Digoxin

31 Bisoprolol

32 Heparin

33 Amlodipine

34 Glyceryl trinitrate (GTN)

35 Indapamide

ANSWERS

TRUE OR FALSE?

1 **Patients with resistant heart failure may experience a marked decrease in blood pressure when angiotensin-converting enzyme (ACE) inhibitors and diuretics are taken concurrently**

This occurs due to the combination of strong vasodilation caused by the ACE inhibitor and reduced circulating blood volume due to the diuretic. The blood pressure of such patients should be regularly monitored, remembering that the onset of hypotension may be delayed for hours with some ACE inhibitors but last up to 36 hours (such as with enalapril).

2 **Lidocaine can be administered orally to reduce cardiac arrthymias**

Lidocaine undergoes significant first-pass metabolism and is therefore not suitable for oral administration. It should be given intravenously. It suppresses excitability in the muscle surrounding the ventricles. Mexiletine has a similar mechanism of action to lignocaine and is particularly useful since it can be administered orally.

3 **Cardioselective beta-blockers target the beta$_2$ adrenoceptors in the myocardium**

Cardioselective beta-blockers such as atenolol predominantly target the beta$_1$ adrenoceptors, which are located mainly in the heart muscle tissue. Beta-blockers may be described as cardioselective or non-cardioselective. *Cardioselective* beta-blockers restrict the binding of adrenaline to beta$_1$ receptors in the heart muscle tissue and have less effect on beta$_2$ receptors lining the respiratory tract. *Non-cardioselective* beta-blockers such as propranolol block both beta$_1$ receptors in the myocardium and beta$_2$ receptors lining the respiratory tract. When adrenaline binds to beta$_2$ receptors bronchodilation is triggered, since these receptors are located on cells lining the bronchi of the lungs; non-cardioselective beta-blockers suppress bronchodilation because the beta$_1$ and beta$_2$ receptors are blocked, thus non-cardioselective beta-blockers are not recommended for patients with respiratory disorders.

4 **Patients with coronary heart disease may be prescribed anticoagulant drugs**

Anticoagulant (or anticlotting) drugs help reduce the risk of blood clots forming in the circulation either by inhibiting the clotting cascade or by interfering with the activity of blood platelets. Warfarin, heparin, and aspirin are examples of anticoagulant drugs that reduce the ability of the blood to clot, although they work in different ways. Warfarin inhibits the action of vitamin K in the body, which is essential for the formation of essential enzymes in the blood coagulation cascade. Heparin prolongs the time taken for a blood clot to form by preventing fibrinogen being converted to fibrin. Aspirin prevents platelets from clumping together (aggregating) to form a clot; hence it is sometimes called an antiplatelet agent. Patients on anticoagulant therapies require frequent monitoring of their blood to ensure they are on the correct dose. The main side-effect associated with anticoagulant drugs is an increased likelihood of prolific bleeding.

5 | **Beta-blockers and calcium channel blockers act as positive inotropes**

Beta-blockers and calcium channel blockers act as negative inotropic drugs because they reduce the workload of the heart by decreasing the rate and the strength of the heartbeat. These effects decrease the volume of blood being pumped by the heart; they also reduce blood pressure in the vessels and the amount of oxygen that the heart requires. The action of these drugs also causes a decrease in electrical activity in the heart. The effects of negative inotropic drugs make them very suitable for treating high blood pressure, angina, and myocardial infarctions (MIs). Their effects on electrical activity make them useful for the treatment of some types of arrhythmias.

6 | **Alpha-adrenoceptor blockers are generally used in combination with other antihypertensive drugs when treating resistant hypertension**

Alpha-adrenoceptor blockers (or alpha-blockers) such as prazosin and doxazosin are generally used to treat resistant hypertension in combination with other antihypertensives rather than on their own as single-agent therapy. The sympathetic nervous system releases the neurotransmitters adrenaline and noradrenaline that bind to alpha$_1$ receptors of arterioles causing vasoconstriction. Vascular smooth muscle has two primary types of alpha-adrenoceptors: alpha$_1$ and alpha$_2$. Alpha$_1$ adrenoceptors are located on the vascular smooth muscle while alpha$_2$ adrenoceptors are located on the sympathetic nerve terminals as well as on vascular smooth muscle. Blocking alpha$_1$ receptors results in relaxation of the smooth muscles of the arterioles, causing vasodilation and hence reducing hypertension.

7 | **Nitrate drugs act directly on all the involuntary muscles of the body causing them to relax**

Nitrates work in one of two ways: (1) they widen the arteries that carry blood to the heart muscle, or (2) they relax the veins that return blood from the body to the heart. The action of nitrates is particularly strong on the muscular walls of the arteries and veins. There are a number of drugs in the nitrate group that vary according to the strength of their action and the duration of action: some are powerful but have a short-lived action, such as sublingual glyceryl trinitrate (GTN), while others are less powerful but have a longer duration of action, such as sustained-release isosorbide dinitrate or isosorbide mononitrate. Sublingual GTN is one of the most effective drugs for providing rapid relief of angina symptoms; an aerosol alternative is available for patients who have difficulty in dissolving sublingual preparations. GTN and isosorbide dinitrate may be administered by IV injection when the sublingual preparation is insufficient, such as in chest pain due to MI or severe ischaemia. Isosorbide mononitrate will not treat an angina attack that has already begun.

8 | Methyldopa lowers blood pressure by acting on parasympathetic nervous activity in the brain

Methyldopa is a central sympathetic inhibitor that lowers blood pressure by stimulating alpha$_2$ receptors in the brain to reduce secretion of the neurotransmitter noradrenaline. Methyldopa is converted to methylnoradrenaline, which inhibits the action of noradrenaline on blood vessels and also lowers arterial blood pressure and heart rate. Methyldopa has a number of adverse effects, including drowsiness and depression, although these can be minimized if the daily dose is under 1 g. It is safe to use when treating hypertension in pregnancy. Clonidine, which is a central sympathetic inhibitor but in addition has a peripheral action on arteries, is not recommended for use in pregnancy or breastfeeding.

9 | Anticoagulant drugs can be used to prevent and treat an arterial or venous thrombosis

Obstruction due to thrombosis may occur in any vessel, although the causes and treatments differ according to their location. Venous thrombosis tends to occur in the deep veins of the legs and is due to stagnation of blood in the veins while immobilized (after surgery or on a long-haul flight). Anticoagulant drugs (such as heparin) may be prescribed to prevent formation of thrombi (while immobilized) or to treat established venous thrombosis. Warfarin is usually the treatment of choice for established venous thrombosis. Arterial thrombosis is associated with increasing age and development of atheroma in the lining of the arterial vessels, which can form a plaque that platelets can stick to and block the vessel. Thrombolytic agents may be used to break down the clot and unblock the artery; however, to be successful, this treatment must be commenced within 24 hours of symptom onset. Antiplatelet drugs (a form of anticoagulant) can be prescribed to prevent platelets from aggregating (sticking together), thus reducing the risk of platelets forming a thrombus. Statins may also be recommended to reduce the risk of developing atheroma and hence lower the risk of coronary thrombosis.

MULTIPLE CHOICE

Correct answers identified in bold italics.

10 **Which of the following types of drugs is not normally used to treat cardiac failure?**

a) diuretics

b) ACE inhibitors

c) *antiplatelet treatments*

d) positive inotropic drugs

In cardiac failure, the cardiac output is reduced, causing a decreased supply of oxygenated blood to the organs and tissues. This is a particular problem in the kidneys where decreased blood supply leads to insufficient excretion of water and salt in the urine, leading to retention of these substances, causing oedema. There are three main objectives when treating cardiac failure: (1) increase efficiency and output from the heart, (2) reduce oedema, and (3) (where possible) remove the factors causing heart failure. Diuretics are the most important drugs used to treat cardiac failure, since they reduce oedema and cardiac distension. ACE inhibitors dilate blood vessels and lower blood pressure; they also inhibit the hormone aldosterone and hence reduce retention of water and salt by the body. Positive inotropic drugs increase the force of cardiac muscle contraction, making the myocardium contraction stronger and thus increasing cardiac output; they include the cardiac glycosides digoxin and digitoxin (of which digoxin is more commonly used for treatment of heart failure). Antiplatelet drugs are a form of anticoagulant therapy prescribed to reduce platelet aggregation in the arterial circulation. They are not part of treatment for heart failure.

11 **Verapamil, used to treat hypertension, angina, and certain arrhythmias, is classified as which type of drug?**

a) beta-blocker

b) ACE inhibitor

c) cardiac glycoside

d) *calcium channel blocker*

Verapamil is a calcium channel blocker, since it inhibits the movement of calcium ions into the cells of the myocardium; this reduces the force of contraction of the myocardium and slows conduction of electrical signals. It is particularly useful in supraventricular tachycardia, as it breaks the circus wave of electrical stimulation between the atrioventricular node and the bundle of His. Calcium channel blockers exert their effects by different mechanisms: (1) on the specialized cells of the heart's electrical conduction tissue, which reduces heart rate; (2) on the cells of the myocardium to reduce stroke volume; and (3) on the smooth muscles of the arterioles to reduce systemic vascular resistance.

12 **Which of the following types of drug would not be used to treat cardiac arrhythmias?**

a) *ACE inhibitors*

b) beta-blockers

c) cardiac glycosides

d) calcium channel blockers

There are many types and causes of cardiac arrhythmias: some are defined by abnormal heart rates (tachycardia and bradycardia), while others are due to abnormal electrical signals in the myocardium. Treatment of arrhythmias aims to restore normal rhythms and the drugs used will depend on the type of arrhythmia. Beta-blockers (such as propranolol and atenolol) block the beta$_1$ adrenoceptors in the myocardial tissue and hence the effects of adrenaline and noradrenaline are inhibited, causing a decrease in myocardial contraction and reduction in heart rate. Cardiac glycosides (such as digoxin) increase the concentration of calcium ions in the heart cells (myocytes); this slows the heart rate and increases the force of contraction of the myocardium. Calcium channel blockers (such as verapamil) block the calcium ion channels in the myocytes, which reduces the concentration of calcium in the conducting tissue, thus slowing the heart rate and reducing the force of contraction.

13 **ACE inhibitor drugs lower blood pressure by targeting which enzyme system?**

a) coagulation cascade   *b)* *renin-angiotensin system*
c) complement system   d) digestive enzymes

ACE inhibitors target the powerful vasoconstricting action triggered by the renin-angiotensin system (RAS) (Figure 7.1). ACE inhibitors prevent conversion of the enzyme angiotensin I into angiotensin II. ACE inhibitors block angiotensin-converting enzymes, so circulating concentrations of angiotensin II are reduced (see Figure 7.1). This results in less vaso-constriction and lower concentrations of sodium in the blood, which reduces blood volume and preload and therefore lowers blood pressure. The side-effects of ACE inhibitors include hypotension, especially in patients who also take diuretics. Persistent dry cough is also a common side-effect associated with ACE inhibitors, although this can be overcome by prescribing angiotensin II receptor antagonists. These drugs do not inhibit activation of angiotensin II but instead block angiotensin receptors in the vasculature and therefore reduce the vasoconstrictive effect of circulating angiotensin II.

14 **Furosemide, which can be used to treat congestive cardiac failure, acts on which part of the kidneys?**

a) nephron   b) proximal convoluted tubule
c) *loop of Henlé*   d) distal convoluted tubule

Furosemide is a loop diuretic that acts on the loop of Henlé, blocking the transport of sodium, potassium, and chloride ions. This interferes with the sodium balance in the kidney, resulting in less water being reabsorbed from the filtrate and more urine being produced. Since sodium reabsorption is inhibited, loop diuretics can result in considerable loss of sodium in the urine. The adverse side-effects of loop diuretics include hyponatraemia, hypokalaemia, and hypomagnesia.

Figure 7.1 The effects of ACE inhibitors and angiotensin II antagonists on the renin-angiotensin system

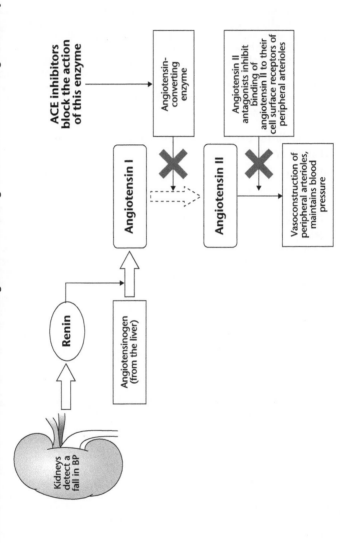

15 | Patients on long-acting or transdermal nitrate formulations can rapidly develop:

a) tolerance   b)   toxicity   c)   adverse reaction   d)   drowsiness

Patients on long-acting or transdermal nitrate formulations can rapidly develop tolerance, which can easily be reversed and sensitivity restored by reducing blood nitrate concentrations to low levels for 4–8 hours each day. If tolerance is suspected when using transdermal nitrate patches, the patch should be left off for several consecutive hours in each 24-hour period. For patients using modified-release isosorbide dinitrate tablets, the second of the two daily doses should be taken after 8 hours rather than after 12 hours. GTN is unlikely to produce tolerance because it is very short-acting.

16 | In the treatment of shock, noradrenaline primarily acts on which adrenergic receptors?

a) $beta_2$ adrenoceptor   　　b) $beta_1$ adrenoceptor

c) $alpha_2$ adrenoceptor   　　*d) $alpha_1$ adrenoceptor*

Noradrenaline acts as a sympathomimetic agent, raising blood pressure by increasing contraction of the muscular vessel walls through activation of $alpha_1$ adrenergic receptors. Constriction of blood vessels increases vascular resistance, which triggers a compensatory reflex that overcomes the baroreceptor reflex, which otherwise would result in bradycardia.

17 | How do statins work to lower serum cholesterol concentrations?

a)   prevent absorption of saturated fats from the diet

b)   inhibit an enzyme involved in production of cholesterol by the body

c)   prevent storage of excess dietary fats

d)   inhibit glucagon secretion

Cholesterol has an essential role in maintaining normal structure and function of the body's cells. The liver is capable of making endogenous cholesterol through a series of chemical reactions. Statins inhibit a liver enzyme (HMG CoA reductase) that is involved in the production of endogenous cholesterol by the body, thus reducing the amount of endogenous cholesterol synthesized in the body. Despite the reduction in endogenous cholesterol, cells still need a supply of cholesterol, so the liver uses low-density lipoprotein (LDL) cholesterol (so-called 'bad' cholesterol) from the circulating blood to synthesize the cholesterol needed by the body, thereby reducing serum LDL cholesterol in the blood.

18 | Aspirin is classified as an antiplatelet drug. How does it work?

a)   stimulates aggregation of platelets

b)   inhibits formation of platelets

c)   inhibits binding of platelets to fibrin

d)   inhibits breakdown of platelets

Aspirin suppresses the activation of platelets by irreversibly inhibiting the COX-1 enzyme, which prevents the synthesis of a prostaglandin required to form fibrin-binding receptors on platelets. This prevents the platelets from expressing receptors necessary to bind with fibrin. If the platelets do not bind with fibrin, a clot cannot form, thus inhibiting coagulation of blood.

FILL IN THE BLANKS

19 *Diuretics* **are the most important drugs for relieving cardiac failure.**

Diuretics reduce peripheral oedema and the associated preload congestion on the heart by increasing the secretion of water and salt by the kidneys. This decreases blood volume and cardiac filling pressure. The reduced distension allows the heart to work more efficiently and alleviates the dyspnoea associated with heart failure. Thiazides and loop diuretics are both suitable, although loop diuretics are more powerful than thiazides but have a shorter duration of action. Both types of diuretics increase the excretion of potassium ions by the kidneys into the urine and a potassium supplement is often necessary to prevent excessive loss of potassium. Supplementary potassium is particularly important if the patient is concurrently prescribed a cardiac glycoside (such as digoxin), since a deficiency in potassium increases the toxicity of cardiac glycosides.

20 *Beta-blockers* **may be prescribed to reduce hypertension.**

Beta-blockers block the effects of the sympathetic nervous system on the heart, which reduces cardiac output, although they may take weeks to produce this effect. Some beta-blockers (particularly propranolol) can have a sedative effect. The precise mechanism of action of beta-blockers is not well understood.

21 **Drugs that increase the lumen of arterioles are called** *vasodilators*.

Vasodilators open up (dilate) arterioles and therefore reduce peripheral resistance in the systemic vasculature. This reduces preload and afterload on the heart and cardiac output increases. ACE inhibitors are widely used vasodilators that decrease the afterload on the heart by inhibiting the conversion of angiotensin I to angiotensin II, which decreases vasoconstriction and decreases aldosterone secretion (see Figure 7.1).

22 **Non-selective beta-blockers are contra-indicated for patients with certain** *respiratory* **conditions.**

Ideally, patients who have a history of asthma or bronchospasm should avoid all beta-blockers, as they inhibit bronchodilation. In cases where there is no suitable alternative to a beta-blocker, then a selective beta-blocker such as atenolol may be used with extreme caution under specialist supervision. Although selective beta-blockers are cardioselective, they are not cardiac specific and while they preferentially target beta$_1$ receptors in the myocardium, they still have a reduced effect on beta$_2$ receptors found in the respiratory airways.

23 | ***Sympathomimetics* are used in the treatment of shock to improve tissue perfusion.**

Adrenaline is a sympathomimetic used in the treatment of shock to improve tissue perfusion. It does not maintain blood pressure. Vasodilators are also used for the treatment of shock often when the systemic shock is due to cardiac failure following acute MI. The vasodilator will relieve preload and afterload as well as limiting the ischaemic damage by increasing the oxygen supply to myocardial tissue. Vasodilators that target arteries and veins are more effective in the treatment of shock than vasodilators that primarily target arteries.

24 | ***Adenosine* is usually the treatment of choice for terminating supraventricular tachycardia.**

Adenosine restores normal sinus rhythm by suppressing conduction of electrical signals through the atrioventricular node. It has a very short half-life (8–10 seconds) and most side-effects, such as chest pain, dyspnoea, and pain at site of injection, are short-lived. It is administered by rapid IV injection into a central or large peripheral vein.

25 | **In emergencies such as myocardial infarction, *thrombolytic* agents may be administered to disperse a clot.**

A blood clot (thrombus) may form in the coronary arteries causing a blockage that can lead to myocardial infarction due to the reduced blood supply to the heart. In such cases, thrombolytic (fibrinolytic) drugs may be administered to the patient to lyse (break down) the thrombus and restore blood and oxygen supply to the affected myocardial tissue. Thrombolytic drugs stimulate the natural clot-inhibiting enzyme, plasmin, to degrade the insoluble fibrin in the thrombus (see Figure 7.2); therefore, thrombolytic drugs mimic the action and are structurally similar to the natural protein, tissue plasminogen activator (t-PA). To be effective, thrombolytic agents must be administered as soon as possible after symptoms develop. The sooner treatment is commenced, the better the outcome for the patient.

26 | **Iron-deficiency anaemia is characterized by a low *haemoglobin* concentration.**

Although there are a number of types of anaemia, iron deficiency is the most common. Other forms of anaemia may be caused by a lack of vitamin B$_{12}$ or folate in the body. Iron deficiency develops when there is an inadequate supply of iron in the body, which is required to synthesize haemoglobin. If haemoglobin concentrations are low, the oxygen-carrying capacity of the blood is reduced. Iron-deficiency anaemia can be caused by a number of things: blood loss, increased demand for iron in the body

Figure 7.2 Clot-busting mechanism of thrombolytic drugs

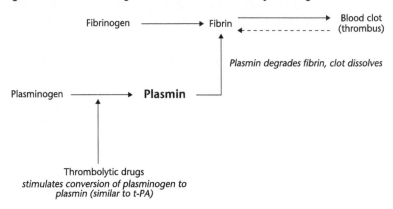

(during growth or pregnancy), decreased absorption of iron from the diet or insufficient dietary intake of iron. The condition is diagnosed from a full blood count, which indicates a lower than normal level of haemoglobin (this varies with gender). Iron-deficiency anaemia is usually treated with oral iron supplements, which should restore haemoglobin concentrations within three months, if the iron is properly absorbed. Often patients are recommended to take iron supplements with a drink of orange juice, since the vitamin C in orange juice increases the absorption of iron by the GI tract. This is an example of a useful drug–food interaction.

MATCH THE TERMS

27	Fosinopril sodium	**I.** ACE inhibitor
28	Reteplase	**B.** thrombolytic (fibrinolytic)
29	Simvastatin	**G.** lipid regulator
30	Digoxin	**E.** positive inotrope
31	Bisoprolol	**C.** cardioselective beta-blocker
32	Heparin	**A.** anticoagulant
33	Amlodipine	**F.** calcium channel blocker
34	Glyceryl trinitrate (GTN)	**H.** antiangina (short-acting)
35	Indapamide	**D.** antihypertensive (thiazide diuretic)

Figure 7.3 Drugs used to treat cardiovascular disorders

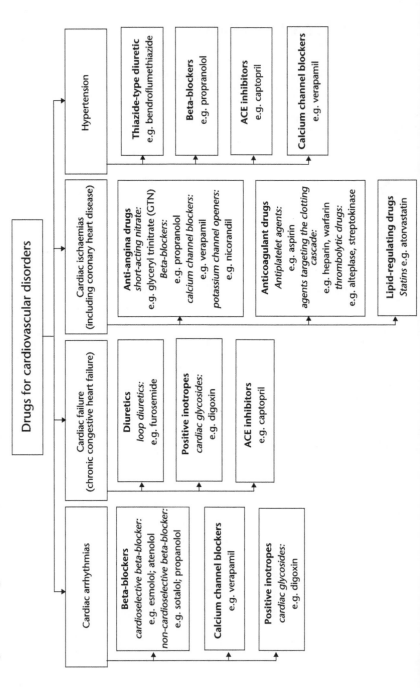

8 Drugs and the respiratory system

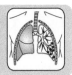

INTRODUCTION

The respiratory system is responsible for the exchange of oxygen and carbon dioxide between tissues, blood, and the external environment. The normal functioning of the lungs is vital for maintaining homeostasis in the body. Many acute and chronic respiratory diseases can reduce the capacity of the respiratory system to adequately facilitate gas exchange and this can quickly disrupt normal physiological homeostasis throughout the body.

Common respiratory conditions that often require pharmacological treatment include asthma, chronic obstructive pulmonary diseases (emphysema and chronic bronchitis), allergies, coughs, and bacterial infections of the respiratory tract. Drug therapy may be required to treat conditions or to alleviate symptoms by fighting infection, reducing inflammation or dilating the airways. Inhalation is a useful route of administration when treating disorders of the respiratory tract, since it gets to the desired site of action very quickly and usually causes fewer side-effects than oral or systemic routes.

Nurses are often responsible for monitoring a patient's oxygen and carbon dioxide levels, so it is important that they are able to recognize and understand the pharmacology of drugs used to treat respiratory conditions. They must be able to teach patients how to take their medication effectively (especially if using inhalers) and they need to know about the adverse effects associated with respiratory drugs.

Useful resources

Nurses! Test Yourself in Essential Calculation Skills
Chapters 1 and 2

Nurses! Test Yourself in Anatomy and Physiology
Chapter 8

Essentials of Pharmacology for Nurses, 2nd edition
Chapter 7

TRUE OR FALSE?

Are the following statements true or false?

1 Bronchodilator drugs specifically target the beta$_2$ adrenoceptors to open up the airways.

2 Antimuscarinic drugs can be prescribed to stimulate bronchodilation.

3 High doses of expectorant medicines can have an antiemetic effect.

4 Aminophylline is a mixture of theophylline and ethylenediamine.

5 Spacer devices are useful for patients with poor inhalation technique when using inhalers.

a b c d MULTIPLE CHOICE

Identify one correct answer for each of the following.

6 The most effective bronchodilator drugs are:

a) antimuscarinics

b) beta$_1$ agonists

c) beta$_2$ agonists

d) theophylline

7 Which of the following drugs is a short-acting beta$_2$ agonist?

a) salbutamol

b) salmeterol

c) ipratropium bromide

d) beclomethasone dipropionate

8 Which of the following statements is incorrect when considering inhalation as a route of administration for asthma drugs?

a) drug is delivered directly to the site of action in the airways

b) required dose is lower than given orally

c) side-effects are more marked

d) solutions may be nebulized for acute severe asthma

9 Which of the following drug types should be used to reduce inflammation of the airways?

a) antimuscarinics

b) bronchodilators

c) antibiotics

d) corticosteroids

10 Leukotriene receptor antagonists are effective in the prophylaxis of which respiratory condition?

a) emphysema

b) exercise-induced asthma

c) cough

d) bronchiectasis

FILL IN THE BLANKS

Fill in the blanks in each statement using the options in the box below.
Not all of them are required, so choose carefully!

salbutamol	gas
antimuscarinic	aerosol
antihistamines	theophylline
anti-inflammatory	antibacterials

11 Ipratropium bromide is an _____ bronchodilating drug.

12 _____ is a bronchodilator used in the treatment of asthma and stable COPD.

13 A nebulizer converts a solution of a drug into an _____ for inhalation.

14 _____ provide relief from nasal allergies, including hayfever.

15 Bacterial respiratory infections such as pneumonia can usually be treated with _____.

MATCH THE TERMS

Match each of the drugs with the listed pharmacological/clinical functions:

A. compound bronchodilator

B. anti-inflammatory

C. short-acting beta2 agonist

D. antimuscarinic

E. antitussive (cough suppressant)

F. corticosteroid

G. antihistamine

H. leukotriene receptor antagonist

I. allergic emergencies

J. long-acting beta2 agonist

---

16 Ipratropium bromide

17 Bambuterol

18 Formeterol

19 Beclometasone diproprionate

20 Cetirizine hydrochloride

21 Roflumilast

22 Intramuscular adrenaline

23 Pholcodeine linctus

24 Ipratropium and salbutamol

25 Montelukast

ANSWERS

TRUE OR FALSE?

1 | **Bronchodilator drugs specifically target the beta$_2$ adrenoceptors to open up the airways**

Bronchodilators are either short acting or longer acting. Short-acting medications provide quick relief from acute bronchoconstriction. Longer-acting bronchodilators help to control and prevent symptoms. There are three types of prescription bronchodilating drugs: (1) selective beta$_2$ agonists (or beta$_2$ adrenergic receptor agonists) that can be short acting or longer acting; (2) antimuscarinics; and (3) theophylline and aminophylline.

Beta$_1$ adrenoceptors are predominantly located in the heart, whereas beta$_2$ adrenoceptors are primarily found in the blood vessels and bronchioles. A bronchodilator dilates the bronchi and bronchioles, opening up the air passages, decreasing resistance in the respiratory airway and increasing airflow to the lungs. Bronchodilators may be endogenous (originating naturally within the body) or medications administered for the treatment of breathing difficulties. They are most useful in obstructive lung diseases, of which asthma and chronic obstructive pulmonary disease (COPD) are the most common conditions.

2 | **Antimuscarinic drugs can be prescribed to stimulate bronchodilation**

Antimuscarinics stimulate bronchodilation but have a slower onset of action than beta$_2$ agonists. They are less effective in the treatment of asthma when inhaled, but are equally as effective when inhaled as treatment for COPD. Ipratropium can provide short-term relief of bronchoconstriction in asthma, although short-acting beta$_2$ agonists act more quickly and are therefore preferred. Tiotropium is a longer-acting antimuscarinic bronchodilator and is therefore not effective in relieving acute bronchospasm. It is recommended for the management of COPD.

3 | **High doses of expectorant medicines can have an antiemetic effect**

Expectorants are drugs often prescribed for a cough that loosen sputum, aiding its expulsion from the respiratory tract. If a large dose is taken, they can have an emetic (vomit-inducing) effect. They often contain a mixture of pseudoephedrine, which induces vasoconstriction to clear nasal congestion, codeine and antihistamines, both of which have antitussive effects (suppresses cough).

4 | **Aminophylline is a mixture of theophylline and ethylenediamine**

Aminophylline is a stable combination of theophylline and ethylenediamine and is used when injection of theophylline is required. Aminophylline is 20 times more soluble than theophylline alone, with the ethylenediamine providing greater solubility in water. Aminophylline must be administered very slowly by IV injection (over at least 20 minutes); it is too much of an irritant for intramuscular injection. Plasma theophylline concentrations should be measured because serious side-effects such as convulsions and arrhythmias may occur.

5 | **Spacer devices are useful for patients with poor inhalation technique when using inhalers**

Some patients, particularly children and older adults, find it difficult to self-administer drugs through inhaler devices. Instead, a spacer device can be used, which removes the need to coordinate the activation of the inhaler with inhalation of the drug. The spacer device reduces the speed of the aerosol expelled during actuation of the inhaler, allowing more time for evaporation of the propellant so that a larger amount of drug is inhaled into the lungs. Spacer devices should not be considered interchangeable, thus it is important that compatible spacer devices are prescribed with the relevant inhalers.

MULTIPLE CHOICE

Correct answers identified in bold italics.

6 | **The most effective bronchodilator drugs are:**

a) antimuscarinics   b) beta$_1$ agonists

c) ***beta$_2$ agonists***   d) theophylline

Selective beta$_2$ agonists are the most effective bronchodilator drugs and are commonly used in the treatment of asthma and certain forms of COPD. They are frequently administered by inhalation, which makes them very effective at quickly relieving acute symptoms such as dyspnoea caused by bronchodilation. They may be used regularly to prevent attacks occurring, although this continued use might lead to the development of drug tolerance. Although oral formulations of the drugs are available, they are most effective and more specific when inhaled. Beta$_2$ agonists are contra-indicated in patients with a history of tachycardia. Selective beta$_2$ agonists work by mimicking the action of adrenaline in the sympathetic nervous system, causing the smooth muscle lining the bronchioles to relax and therefore bronchioles dilate, which facilitates the movement of air through the airways. Antimuscarinic drugs have a slower onset of bronchodilation and are therefore less suitable for acute episodes for asthma. Beta$_1$ agonists selectively target the beta$_1$ adrenergic receptors located in cardiac tissue. Therefore, these drugs act more selectively on the heart and are sometimes called cardioselective beta-blockers (see Chapter 7, Answer 3). Theophylline is less effective as a bronchodilator than beta$_2$ agonists.

7 **Which of the following drugs is a short-acting beta$_2$ agonist?**

a) *salbutamol*   b) salmeterol
c) ipratropium bromide   d) beclomethasone dipropionate

Salbutamol is a popular and effective short-acting beta$_2$ agonist that has a rapid onset when inhaled to quickly relieve bronchoconstriction; it may be used to treat mild-to-moderate symptoms that respond rapidly when treated via inhalation. Salmeterol is a longer-acting beta$_2$ agonist that has a slower onset of action than short-acting drugs but its action is more prolonged (6–12 hours with certain drugs). Longer-acting drugs are delivered by inhalation and used for long-term control of respiratory conditions, alongside regular corticosteroid treatment. Ipratropium bromide is a bronchodilator but not a beta$_2$ agonist; it is an antimuscarinic drug. Beclomethasone dipropionate is an inhaled corticosteroid that may be used in the prophylactic management of asthma.

8 **Which of the following statements is incorrect when considering inhalation as a route of administration for asthma drugs?**

a) drug is delivered directly to the site of action in the airways
b) required dose is lower than given orally
c) *side-effects are more marked*
d) solutions may be nebulized for acute severe asthma

Administering drugs to treat respiratory conditions by inhalation is a very effective route because it allows rapid delivery of drugs to the desired site of action – that is, the respiratory airways. Inhaled drugs do not undergo first-pass metabolism before reaching the lungs and therefore the required dose is usually lower than when giving the drug orally. Side-effects are usually less marked because the drug is being administered to the desired site of action without having to travel in the bloodstream. Treatments may be nebulized in acute severe cases. When nebulization is not possible or inadequate, beta$_2$ agonists, corticosteroids, and aminophylline may be given by injection. Beta$_2$ agonists, corticosteroids, theophylline, and leukotriene receptor agonists may be given orally when inhalation is not possible.

9 **Which of the following drug types should be used to reduce inflammation of the airways?**

a) antimuscarinics   b) bronchodilators
c) antibiotics   d) *corticosteroids*

Corticosteroids (steroids) are effective in treating asthma and COPD as they reduce inflammation of the airways and hence reduce secretion of mucus in the respiratory tract. Regular use of inhaled corticosteroids reduces the risk of exacerbation of asthma and COPD. Smoking reduces the effectiveness of inhaled corticosteroids, so smokers require higher doses.

Inhaled corticosteroids have fewer side-effects than oral formulations. Systemic treatment may be required during episodes of infection or airways obstruction and hydrocortisone injection may be used to treat acute severe asthma.

10 **Leukotriene receptor antagonists are effective in the prophylaxis of which respiratory condition?**

a) emphysema

b) *exercise-induced asthma*

c) cough

d) bronchiectasis

Exercise-induced asthma occurs when the airways narrow due to exercise. (The more correct term is 'exercise-induced bronchoconstriction' because exercise does not cause asthma, but is frequently an asthma trigger.) Leukotriene receptor antagonists are used for the prevention of symptoms, but are not suitable for relief of symptoms once they have developed. If asthma symptoms develop despite pre-treatment with leukotriene receptor antagonists, a rapid-acting bronchodilator should be used. Leukotriene receptor antagonists work by reducing airway narrowing, inflammation, and mucus production. Examples of leukotriene modifiers include montelukast and zafirlukast. These are taken orally once daily (montelukast) or twice daily (zafirlukast) and have relatively few side-effects. Taken regularly, either of these medications is useful in preventing exercise-induced bronchospasm.

FILL IN THE BLANKS

11 **Ipratropium bromide is an _antimuscarinic_ bronchodilating drug.**

Ipratropium bromide is an antagonistic antimuscarinic drug that acts as a bronchodilator by competitively blocking the action of the neurotransmitter acetylcholine at the parasympathetic (cholinergic) receptors. Drug tolerance does not appear to be a problem with ipratropium bromide and it does not exhibit the cardiotoxicity associated with selective $beta_2$ agonists; this makes it a good alternative where $beta_2$ agonists are contra-indicated. Beclomethasone dipropionate is an anti-inflammatory corticosteroid that can be inhaled. This makes it a useful corticosteroid, since the adverse effects associated with systemic corticosteroids can be avoided.

12 ***Theophylline* is a bronchodilator used in the treatment of asthma and stable COPD.**

Theophylline is usually ineffective in exacerbations of COPD. There is a considerable variation in the plasma concentrations of theophylline in smokers and in patients with heart failure or hepatic impairment or if drugs are administered concurrently. Differences in the half-life of theophylline are important because its therapeutic dose and its toxic dose are very similar. In most patients, a plasma theophylline concentration of 10–20 mg/litre is required to induce satisfactory bronchodilation, although adverse effects can occur within this range, the frequency and severity of which increase above 20 mg/litre.

13 **A nebulizer converts a solution of a drug into an *aerosol* for inhalation.**

A nebulizer is used to deliver higher doses of drugs into the air passages than can normally be delivered through inhalers. They are often employed to deliver bronchodilators in cases of acute severe asthma or chronic COPD and may also be used to deliver prophylactic corticosteroid to patients (such as children) who are unable to use other inhalation devices. Antibiotics may be delivered by nebulization to patients with chronic purulent infection, such as cystic fibrosis or bronchiectasis. From a nursing perspective, it is important that the patient is aware the doses received by nebulization are much higher than those delivered through an aerosol inhaler.

14 ***Antihistamines* provide relieve from nasal allergies, including hayfever.**

Antihistamines are commonly prescribed to reduce the symptoms associated with nasal allergies, including seasonal allergic rhinitis (hayfever). They reduce discharge of nasal mucus (rhinorrhoea) and sneezing but are usually less effective in reducing nasal congestion. Older antihistamines (such as chlorphenamine, cyclizine, and promethazine) can have a sedating effect because they have significant penetration of the blood–brain barrier; non-sedating antihistamines (cetirizine, loratidine, fexofenazine, and mizolastine) have only slight blood–brain barrier penetration. Side-effects are more common with older antihistamines and include blurred vision, drowsiness, dry mouth, headache, and GI disturbances; less common side-effects include hypotension, arrhythmias, palpitation, dizziness, and anaphylaxis.

15 **Bacterial respiratory infections such as pneumonia can usually be treated with *antibacterials*.**

The most common cause of pneumonia in adults is the bacteria *Streptococcus pneumoniae*. This form of pneumonia is sometimes called pneumococcal pneumonia and is usually successfully treated at home with a course of antibacterial drugs (antibiotics) such as co-amoxiclav prescribed by the GP. Antibiotic treatment usually works for bacterial respiratory infections. If symptoms do not begin to improve within two days of starting treatment, it may be because the bacteria causing the infection are resistant to the antibiotics, in which case the doctor may change to a different antibiotic, or they may prescribe a second antibiotic concurrent with the first one. Alternatively, a virus may be causing the infection, rather than bacteria, and antibiotics will have no effect on viruses. Some patients may need hospital treatment if their symptoms are severe or they have a compromised immune system.

MATCH THE TERMS

16 Ipratropium bromide **D.** antimuscarinic

17 Bambuterol **C.** short-acting beta$_2$ agonist

18 Formeterol **J.** long-acting beta$_2$ agonist

19 Beclometasone diproprionate **F.** corticosteroid

20 Cetirizine hydrochloride **G.** antihistamine

21 Roflumilast **B.** anti-inflammatory

22 Intramuscular adrenaline **I.** allergic emergencies

23 Pholcodeine linctus **E.** antitussive (cough suppressant)

24 Ipratropium and salbutamol **A.** compound bronchodilator

25 Montelukast **H.** leukotriene receptor antagonist

Figure 8.1 Drugs for common disorders of the respiratory system

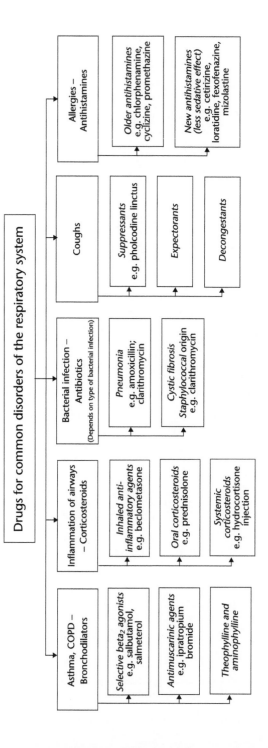

9 Drugs and the digestive system

INTRODUCTION

The digestive – or gastrointestinal (GI) – system consists of a number of primary and accessory organs that collectively process food and absorb nutrients from the diet to maintain a healthy body.

Diseases of the GI system can be localized to a specific organ or may affect various neural and hormonal pathways linked to the system, which can have a significant impact on GI function. Similarly, any imbalance in digestive function can have a serious effect on the other body systems and may significantly reduce quality of life if appropriate treatment is not administered. Common GI complaints include gastro-oesophageal reflux disease (GORD), dyspepsia, ulcers, infection, obstruction, and motility problems.

Many drugs are available without prescription for the treatment of common minor GI conditions, while other conditions require treatment with prescribed medication. Surgery may be preferred for more serious cases, particularly those that may lead to acute or chronic life-threatening conditions. It is important for nurses to be knowledgeable about over-the-counter and prescription drugs that affect the GI system to help alleviate symptoms, reduce potential complications, limit unwanted drug interactions, and prevent exacerbation of conditions due to associated nutritional deficits.

Useful resources

Nurses! Test Yourself in Anatomy and Physiology
Chapter 9

Nurses! Test Yourself in Pathophysiology
Chapter 9

Further Essentials of Pharmacology for Nurses
Chapter 2

Gastrointestinal pharmacology review
http://www.medquarterly.co.uk/mq88/index.php/learning-notes/2012-02-18-18-22-41/mq-pharmacology/article/7-gi-drugs

TRUE OR FALSE?

Are the following statements true or false?

1   *Helicobacter pylori* is a major cause of peptic ulcer.

2   Proton pump inhibitors increase secretion of stomach acid.

3   Compound preparations of antacids and alginates increase stomach pH and reduce symptoms of indigestion.

4   Aluminium-containing antacids tend to have laxative effects, whereas magnesium-containing preparations tend to be constipating.

5   Opioid-related drugs decrease peristalsis within the intestine.

6   A high-fibre diet should be the primary treatment for constipation.

a b c d   MULTIPLE CHOICE

Identify one correct answer for each of the following.

7 A side-effect of some drugs is that they interfere with gastric motility.
Which of the following is not associated with this problem?

a) paracetamol

b) opioids

c) antimuscarinics

d) calcium channel blockers

8 Which of the following is not a form of laxative?

a) bulk-forming laxative

b) osmotic laxative

c) relaxant laxative

d) stimulant laxative

9 Lactulose is contra-indicated in patients with:

a) lactose intolerance

b) intestinal obstruction

c) dehydration

d) gastric cancer

10 Which of the following is not normally found in preparations for treating
haemorrhoids?

a) anti-inflammatory corticosteroid

b) NSAID

c) local anaesthetic

d) mild astringent

11 Which of the following may be used to alleviate the abdominal pain associated with irritable bowel syndrome?

a) paracetamol

b) local anaesthetic

c) NSAID

d) tricyclic antidepressant

12 Gastroenteritis is a common infection of the GI tract that may be caused by bacterial or viral pathogens. Which of the following viruses is not associated with gastroenteritis?

a) norovirus

b) varicella zoster virus

c) rotavirus

d) adenovirus

FILL IN THE BLANKS

Fill in the blanks in each statement using the options in the box below.
Not all of them are required, so choose carefully!

corticosteroids	sulfuric acid
codeine	hydrochloric acid
antimuscarinics	diarrhoea
vomiting	morphine

13 H_2 receptor antagonists block certain histamine receptors and reduce the secretion of _____ _____ in the stomach.

14 A mixture of kaolin and _____ may be prescribed to treat acute diarrhoea.

15 _____ are not suitable as treatment to maintain remission from inflammatory bowel conditions.

16 _____ relax the smooth muscle of the GI tract and can be used to relieve the spasm and pain associated with irritable bowel syndrome and diverticular disease.

17 Antiemetics may be prescribed to alleviate _____.

MATCH THE TERMS

Match each of the drugs with the listed pharmacological/clinical functions:

A. bulk-forming laxative   E. antiemetic

B. proton pump inhibitor   F. antidiarrhoeal

C. osmotic laxative   G. H_2 receptor antagonist

D. antibiotic   H. antiflatulent

---

18 Loperamide   **22** Lansoprazole

19 Metaclopramide   **23** Methylcellulose

20 Simeticone   **24** Clarithromycin

21 Ranitidine   **25** Lactulose

ANSWERS

TRUE OR FALSE?

1   *Helicobacter pylori* **is a major cause of peptic ulcer**

Helicobacter pylori is a strain of bacteria considered a major cause of peptic ulcers and gastritis (inflammation of the stomach lining). Eradicating the bacteria is necessary for ulcer healing and reducing the chance of recurrence. Successful treatment usually involves a 'triple-therapy regimen', which consists of two antibiotics to treat the bacteria in combination with an antisecretory agent such as a proton pump inhibitor or an H_2 receptor antagonist to reduce acid secretions. The antibiotics commonly used to treat *H. pylori* in an initial triple-therapy regimen include clarithromycin and either amoxicillin or metronidazole. This is prescribed for one week, which usually yields eradication in up to 85% of cases. Failure of the treatment often indicates poor compliance or antibiotic resistance. Two-week regimens may offer better eradication rates but often these effects are reduced due to poor compliance by patients. If an ulcer is large or perforated, the antisecretory treatment may be continued for three weeks following the triple-therapy regimen.

2   **Proton pump inhibitors increase secretion of stomach acid**

Proton pump inhibitors (PPIs) decrease secretion of hydrochloric acid (HCl) in the stomach and relieve the symptoms of GORD and dyspepsia. They may also be used to help eradicate *H. pylori*-induced peptic ulcers and are the first choice of treatment for peptic ulcers caused by NSAIDs; they may be prescribed as prophylactic treatment for patients known to be at risk of an NSAID-induced ulcer. Proton pump inhibitors work by inhibiting the secretion (pumping) of hydrogen ions (protons) from the parietal cells into the stomach; this reduces the formation of HCl and reduces the acidic nature of the stomach. Common examples include lansoprazole and omeprazole. They are considered more effective at reducing acid secretions than H_2 receptor antagonists (such as ranitidine). Proton pump inhibitors and H_2 receptor antagonists can mask symptoms of gastric cancer, which should be investigated in patients exhibiting symptoms before prescribing either type of antisecretory medication. It has recently been suggested that PPIs may be effective in improving asthma symptoms since asthma patients who were taking a PPI (for a gastric problem) reported an improvement in their symptoms. The mechanism of how this may happen is not yet understood.

3   **Compound preparations of antacids and alginates increase stomach pH and reduce symptoms of indigestion**

The alkaline compounds found in antacids increase the pH of the stomach contents (chyme), which alleviates the irritating effects of GORD and dyspepsia. Often antacids are available in combination with an alginate that forms a viscous gel (raft complex) that floats on top of the stomach contents forming a barrier that protects the oesophagus and reduces reflux symptoms. To be classified as a 'raft-forming oral suspension', alginates must contain sodium alginate, sodium bicarbonate, and calcium carbonate. A number of well-known compound antacid–alginate preparations are available to buy over-the-counter as tablet and liquid formulations, although not all of these products are classified as raft-forming oral suspensions (in the BNF) because they do not contain all three of the essential ingredients for this classification.

4 | **Aluminium-containing antacids tend to have laxative effects, whereas magnesium-containing preparations tend to be constipating**

Aluminium-containing antacids tend to constipate, whereas magnesium-containing preparations tend to have laxative effects. Preparations containing both aluminium and magnesium may reduce these side-effects, although the acid-neutralizing effect of such preparations is no more effective than that of preparations containing a single antacid. Liquid preparations tend to be more effective at relieving symptoms than tablet versions. Simeticone may be included in certain antacid formulations to reduce flatulence. Antacids should not be taken with other drugs, as they can reduce drug absorption.

5 | **Opioid-related drugs decrease peristalsis within the intestine**

The constipation-inducing side-effect of opioid drugs can be exploited to provide symptomatic relief of acute (non-specific) diarrhoea and chronic diarrhoea associated with inflammatory bowel disease (IBD). This is due to the effect opioid drugs have on the muscles of the GI tract, which reduces intestinal activity thus prolonging transit time of the intestinal contents, which allows more time for water to be absorbed from the faeces. This reduces the volume of the faeces, prevents the excess loss of fluids and electrolytes, and increases the bulk and viscosity of the faeces. Loperamide is an opioid-related antimotility drug that is available without prescription for the treatment of diarrhoea.

6 | **A high-fibre diet should be the primary treatment for constipation**

When patients experience constipation, it is often due to lifestyle- or non-GI-related disorders, thus a diet high in fibre together with adequate fluids (preferably water) and regular exercise should be the treatment of choice to enhance gastric motility and reduce symptoms. There are three main types of laxative medications available, which work in slightly different ways (see Answer 8).

MULTIPLE CHOICE

7 **A side-effect of some drugs is that they interfere with gastric motility. Which of the following is not associated with this problem?**

a) *paracetamol*
b) opioids
c) antimuscarinics
d) calcium channel blockers

Many drugs, including the opioids (such as codeine), antimuscarinics (such as atropine), and calcium channel blockers (such as verapamil) have constipation as a side-effect because they slow down gastric motility. Constipation is not a reported side-effect associated with paracetamol. However, when paracetamol is prescribed with an opioid as a compound analgesic preparation, even a low-dose opioid may be sufficient to induce opioid-like side-effects including constipation. For example, co-codamol 8/500 has 8 mg of codeine present in combination with 500 mg of paracetamol, which is sufficient to induce constipation in some patients.

8 **Which of the following is not a form of laxative?**

a) bulk-forming laxative
b) osmotic laxative
c) *relaxant laxative*
d) stimulant laxative

When pharmacological treatment is required to relieve constipation, three main types of laxative are available to relieve symptoms in slightly different ways. Bulk-forming laxatives are similar to natural dietary fibre and contain insoluble natural and semi-synthetic polysaccharides and cellulose. They increase the faecal matter and stimulate peristalsis; examples include ispaghula, sterculia, and methylcellulose (which may also be used as a faecal softener). Bulk laxatives may be used to treat patients with haemorrhoids, ulcerative colitis, and irritable bowel syndrome (IBS); patients should be encouraged to drink lots of water to prevent intestinal obstruction. Osmotic laxatives increase the water volume in the large intestine, which softens the faeces and increases faecal mass; examples include lactulose and macrogols, as well as magnesium salts, which may be used when rapid evacuation of the colon is required. Stimulant laxatives increase the volume of fluid secreted into the GI tract, which softens the faeces and stimulates gastric motility; examples include senna and bisacodyl. Excessive use of osmotic and stimulant laxatives can result in diarrhoea and hypokalaemia.

9 **Lactulose is contra-indicated in patients with:**

a) *lactose intolerance*
b) intestinal obstruction
c) dehydration
d) gastric cancer

Lactulose is an osmotic laxative used in the treatment of constipation. As lactulose is a semi-synthetic disaccharide that is chemically very similar to the natural disaccharide lactose, this makes it unsuitable for patients who are lactose intolerant. Lactulose makes the GI tract more acidic, which promotes gastric motility thus stimulating peristalsis. It also increases water content and volume of the faeces, making the faeces softer and easier to pass. This makes it suitable for use in very young babies who may experience constipation.

10 **Which of the following is not normally found in preparations for treating haemorrhoids?**

a) anti-inflammatory corticosteroid *b) NSAID*

c) local anaesthetic   d) mild astringent

Haemorrhoid treatments aim to reduce itching, pain, and inflammation and therefore usually contain a combination of ingredients – namely, an anti-inflammatory corticosteroid such as hydrocortisone, a local anaesthetic such as lidocaine, and a mild astringent such as zinc oxide. The treatment is usually administered topically (in a cream or ointment) or via a suppository. These compound preparations should not be used as long-term treatments for haemorrhoids, as they can cause thinning of the skin (atrophy) around the anus. The local anaesthetic in the preparation is usually sufficient to relieve pain, so an additional pain-relieving compound (such as an NSAID) is not usually part of haemorrhoid preparations.

11 **Which of the following may be used to alleviate the abdominal pain associated with irritable bowel syndrome?**

a) paracetamol   b) local anaesthetic

c) NSAID   *d) tricyclic antidepressant*

Low doses of a tricyclic antidepressant (TCA) may be used to relieve the pain associated with IBS when patients have failed to respond to a laxative such as macrogol, anti-spasmodics such as peppermint oil, or antimotility drugs such as loperamide.

12 **Gastroenteritis is a common infection of the GI tract that may be caused by bacterial or viral pathogens. Which of the following viruses is not associated with gastroenteritis?**

a) norovirus   *b) varicella zoster virus*

c) rotavirus   d) adenovirus

The varicella zoster virus is responsible for causing chicken pox and is not associated with gastroenteritis. Norovirus is the virus commonly linked with the 'winter vomiting bug', which produces symptoms of gastroenteritis, including nausea, vomiting, and diarrhoea. Rotavirus, adenovirus, and astrovirus are all viral pathogens that are also known to cause gastroenteritis. The duration of symptoms usually depends on which viral pathogen has caused the illness. The best treatment for gastroenteritis is to rest and drink plenty of fluids, to allow the symptoms to pass, rather than to take antiemetic and/or antidiarrhoeal medication. This enables the GI tract to purge itself of the damaging pathogen.

Care should be taken in children (particularly babies) and older adults to ensure they do not become dehydrated, which may require hospital admission. Bacterial pathogens, namely *Campylobacter, Salmonella*, and *Escherichia*, can also cause gastroenteritis and induce symptoms that require the same treatment.

FILL IN THE BLANKS

13 **H_2 receptor antagonists block certain histamine receptors and reduce the secretion of _hydrochloric acid_ in the stomach.**

When the neurotransmitter histamine binds to H_2 receptors on the parietal cells lining the stomach, these cells secrete HCl. H_2 receptor antagonist drugs block the H_2 receptors and therefore prevent histamine from binding. This prevents the cells from secreting HCl, making the stomach less acidic and relieving the symptoms of GORD or dyspepsia. Common H_2 receptor antagonists include ranitidine, famotidine, and cimetidine. Cimetidine is not recommended for patients taking warfarin, phenytoin or aminophylline, as it is known to inhibit cytochrome P450 enzymes (which affects metabolism of these drugs) in the liver and elevates serum concentrations of the drugs. The other common H_2 receptor antagonists do not appear to cause this type of drug interaction.

14 **A mixture of kaolin and _morphine_ may be prescribed to treat acute diarrhoea.**

A mixture of kaolin and morphine has antimotility properties that can be used to treat uncomplicated, acute diarrhoea. Kaolin is a type of clay that retains moisture, so the compound increases the viscosity of the faeces being formed in the colon. Morphine (since it is an opioid) slows peristalsis, which enables reabsorption of water and salts from the colon. This helps to form stools, which are firmer and are passed less frequently.

15 **_Corticosteroids_ are not suitable as treatment to maintain remission from inflammatory bowel conditions.**

Despite their anti-inflammatory properties, corticosteroids (steroids) are not suitable as a maintenance treatment for irritable bowel disorder (IBD) due to their side-effects. Aminosalicylates are recommended for maintenance of remission in ulcerative colitis patients but not for Crohn's disease. Instead, azathioprine or mercaptopurine may be given to Crohn's disease patients to maintain remission. Infliximab may be considered as a maintenance treatment in Crohn's disease patients who respond to initial treatment with infliximab. Corticosteroids such as prednisolone may be used to treat acute episodes of IBDs such as Crohn's disease and ulcerative colitis. Patients with IBDs should be educated on the importance of diet in helping to relieve symptoms and maintain remission.

16 ***Antimuscarinics*** **relax the smooth muscle of the GI tract and can be used to relieve the spasm and pain associated with irritable bowel syndrome and diverticular disease.**

Antimuscarinics inhibit the action of the neurotransmitter acetylcholine, which causes the smooth muscle lining the GI tract to relax, reducing gastric motility. This property makes them useful in treating irritable bowel syndrome (IBS) and diverticular disease. Common antimuscarinics used to treat spasm in the smooth muscle of the GI tract include atropine and hyosine butylbromide. Other antispasmodic treatments (that are not antimuscarinic in nature) may also be used to relax the smooth muscle of the GI tract and relieve the pain associated with IBS and diverticular disease; these include alverine, mebeverine, and peppermint oil, and although these have no known adverse effects, peppermint oil can induce heartburn.

17 **Antiemetics may be prescribed to alleviate *vomiting*.**

Antiemetics should only be administered when the cause of the vomiting is known and the drug should be chosen in accordance with this knowledge. They are not routinely prescribed for nausea and vomiting associated with gastroenteritis as their use can delay recovery, since the vomiting reflex is actually helpful in expelling the pathogen causing the illness. When treating nauseas and vomiting associated with motion sickness, antiemetics should be taken before symptoms arise to prevent them developing; often they are ineffective if taken after symptoms present. Most antiemetics, such as $5HT_3$ receptor antagonists (ondansetron), metoclopramide, and phenothiazines (chlorpromazine), act on various parts of the central nervous system rather than directly on the GI system.

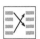 **MATCH THE TERMS**

18 Loperamide   **F.** antidiarrhoeal

19 Metaclopramide   **E.** antiemetic

20 Simeticone   **H.** antiflatulent

21 Ranitidine   **G.** H_2 receptor antagonist

22 Lansoprazole   **B.** proton pump inhibitor

23 Methylcellulose   **A.** bulk-forming laxative

24 Clarithromycin   **D.** antibiotic

25 Lactulose   **C.** osmotic laxative

Figure 9.1 Drugs for common disorders of the digestive system

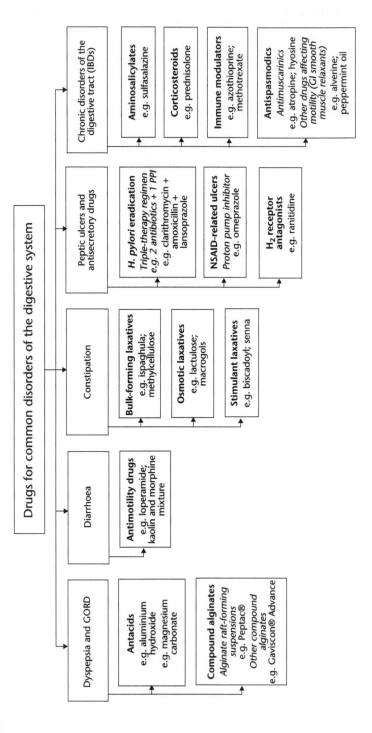

10 Drugs and the urinary system

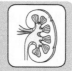

INTRODUCTION

The urinary system (renal system) consists of two kidneys, two ureters, a urinary bladder, and urethra. Its function is to filter the blood, removing waste and toxins and produce, store, and eliminate liquid waste from the body in the form of urine.

The function of the urinary system declines with age but can also be affected by illness or injury. As the body ages, the kidneys' ability to filter blood effectively can decline, while the muscles of the ureters, bladder, and urethra may lose strength. Infections of the urinary tract may become more frequent, since the bladder muscles are weakened and less able to contract sufficiently to fully empty the bladder during urination (micturition). Incontinence can become a problem if the bladder sphincter muscles lose their strength causing leakage of urine. At any age, illness or injury can prevent the kidneys from filtering the blood completely or block the passage of urine through the system.

Conditions affecting the urinary system can be acute or chronic and if not treated immediately, some can become life-threatening. Common conditions include urinary tract infections (UTIs), formation of renal calculi (kidney stones), proteinuria, and urinary retention. Treatment of conditions affecting other organ systems may involve pharmacological manipulation of kidney function, such as treatment of hypertension using diuretic drugs or angiotensin-converting enzyme (ACE) inhibitors. Knowledge of the drugs used to treat these conditions, together with their potential interactions, is essential so that nurses can make informed judgements about patient care and management.

Useful resources

Nurses! Test Yourself in Anatomy and Physiology
Chapter 10

Nurses! Test Yourself in Pathophysiology
Chapter 10

Medications used to treat diseases of the urinary system
http://www.netdoctor.co.uk/medicines/effect/liver_kidney_urinary.shtml

TRUE OR FALSE?

Are the following statements true or false?

1 Males are more susceptible to urinary tract infections than females.

2 NSAIDs are not recommended as painkillers when treating upper urinary tract infections.

3 Antimuscarinic drugs are contra-indicated in patients with significant bladder outflow obstruction or urinary retention.

4 The drug desmopressin is a synthetic analogue of antidiuretic hormone.

5 Diuretics are drugs used to decrease urine output.

6 Aldosterone antagonists enhance the action of the hormone aldosterone on the distal convoluted tubule.

MULTIPLE CHOICE

Identify one correct answer for each of the following.

7 Which of the following is not a type of diuretic?

a) loop diuretic

b) osmotic diuretic

c) sodium-sparing diuretic

d) thiazide diuretic

8 Which of the following natural fruit juices is often recommended for the prevention and treatment of urinary tract infections?

a) cranberry

b) grapefruit

c) lemon

d) tomato

9 Which of the following salt solutions may be used to relieve the symptoms of a mild urinary tract infection?

a) sodium chloride

b) calcium chloride

c) potassium citrate

d) magnesium nitrate

10 The best way of monitoring the effectiveness of a diuretic is by recording:

a) a fluid balance chart

b) weight and height

c) height

d) weight

11 Which of the following is not a form of urinary incontinence?

  a) overflow incontinence

  b) impatient incontinence

  c) stress incontinence

  d) urge incontinence

FILL IN THE BLANKS

Fill in the blanks in each statement using the options in the box below.
Not all of them are required, so choose carefully!

calcium	overflow
thiazides	imipramine
potassium	furosemide
stress	mannitol
loop	clomipramine

12 _____ diuretics are the most potent class of diuretic.

13 _____ is the diuretic of choice for treating cerebral oedema.

14 The electrolyte _____ may be retained as a side-effect of thiazide diuretics.

15 _____ incontinence is the most common type of urinary incontinence.

16 The tricyclic antidepressant _____ may be prescribed to treat nocturnal enuresis in children who have not responded to other treatments.

MATCH THE TERMS

Match each of the drugs with the listed pharmacological/clinical functions:

A. antimuscarinic   F. alkalinizing agent

B. osmotic diuretic   G. aldosterone antagonist

C. loop diuretic   H. antidiuretic

D. thiazide diuretic   I. potassium-sparing diuretic

E. antibiotic

| 17 | Trimethoprim | | 22 | Potassium citrate |

| 18 | Furosemide | | 23 | Amiloride |

| 19 | Oxybutynin | | 24 | Spironolactone |

| 20 | Mannitol | | 25 | Bendroflumethiazide |

| 21 | Desmopressin |

ANSWERS

TRUE OR FALSE?

1 | **Males are more susceptible to urinary tract infections than females**

Females are more susceptible to UTIs than males since the female urethra is closer to the anus and shorter than the male urethra, which enables the pathogen to quickly enter and travel up the urinary tract causing infection. Symptoms of UTIs include pain or burning sensation during urination, lower abdominal pain, a frequent urge to urinate although often expelling very little urine, strong smelling urine, and cloudy or bloody urine. The most common bacteria associated with urinary tract infection is *Escherichia coli*, although *Staphylococcus* infections are also common. Antibiotics are usually prescribed to treat UTIs; the duration of treatment depends on the location of the infection. Lower UTIs (infections of the bladder or urethra) are usually successfully eradicated within a week, while upper UTIs (infection of the ureters or kidneys) may require antibiotics for 7–14 days. Patients should also be advised to consume lots of fluids (preferably water) and painkillers may be used to ease discomfort.

2 | **NSAIDs are not recommended as painkillers when treating upper urinary tract infections**

Over-the-counter painkillers are often required to ease the discomfort of symptoms of upper and lower UTIs. When treating upper UTIs, however, the NSAID family of painkillers (such as ibuprofen and naproxen) are not recommended to relieve symptoms, since these drugs may cause complications to the kidneys which are already under stress from the bacterial infection. In such cases, paracetamol should be used to reduce the pain and fever associated with infection. NSAIDs may be used as pain relief for lower UTIs, since the kidneys are not the site of infection in a lower UTI. Paracetamol is also safe to use as pain relief for a lower UTI.

3 | **Antimuscarinic drugs are contra-indicated in patients with significant bladder outflow obstruction or urinary retention**

Antimuscarinic drugs, such as oxybutynin, are the first line of treatment for an overactive bladder. They work by reducing the involuntary contraction of detrusor muscles – which are smooth muscle fibres lining the wall of the urinary bladder which increases the capacity of the bladder to store more urine. Therefore, these drugs are contra-indicated for patients with a history of urinary retention.

4 | The drug desmopressin is a synthetic analogue of antidiuretic hormone

Desmopressin is very similar to the naturally occurring antidiuretic hormone (ADH or vasopressin), which reduces the output of urine by facilitating more reabsorption of water from the renal filtrate in the distal convoluted tubule and collecting duct; this produces a lower volume of more concentrated urine. Desmopressin has the same effect on the kidneys as ADH, since it reduces the amount of urine produced. It may be administered nasally, intravenously or in tablet form – orally or sublingually. Desmopressin is most frequently prescribed for the treatment of diabetes insipidus, nocturnal enuresis (bedwetting) in adults, and nocturia (passing urine at night). Patients taking desmopressin should be advised not to drink large volumes of fluids, as this can lead to an accumulation of water in the body, which may cause an electrolyte imbalance.

5 | Diuretics are drugs used to decrease urine output

Diuretics are a family of drugs used to increase urine output – for this reason, they are sometimes called 'water tablets'. They are prescribed to treat oedema in a range of disorders, such as heart failure, acute pulmonary oedema, renal disease, and liver cirrhosis. They may also be used to treat hypertension (by reducing blood volume) and cerebral oedema (specifically with mannitol).

6 | Aldosterone antagonists enhance the action of the hormone aldosterone on the distal convoluted tubule

Aldosterone antagonists inhibit the action of aldosterone, which normally triggers the reabsorption of sodium and water but expels potassium into the filtrate at the distal convoluted tubule; examples include spironolactone and eplerenone. Since they act antagonistically (blocking aldosterone receptors), aldosterone antagonists have a mild diuretic action by releasing sodium and water but also have a potassium-sparing effect. They may be prescribed for congestive heart failure, since the excess fluid loss reduces the workload on the heart, and treatment of ascites associated with liver disease. Like other potassium-sparing diuretics, there is a risk of hyperkalaemia. Patients should not take aldosterone antagonists in conjunction with potassium supplements, and care is required in patients also taking ACE inhibitors, as this combination can cause potassium retention by the kidneys.

MULTIPLE CHOICE

Correct answers identified in bold italics.

7 **Which of the following is not a type of diuretic?**

a) loop diuretic   b) osmotic diuretic
c) sodium-sparing diuretic   d) thiazide diuretic

There is no diuretic classified as 'sodium-sparing', although there is a group called potassium-sparing diuretics. They act on the distal convoluted tubule and conserve potassium, meaning they are regularly used with other diuretics, such as loop diuretics, to conserve potassium. However, there is a risk of hyperkalaemia if they are used alone and patients should not take potassium supplements while on this type of diuretic. They should also avoid ingesting large quantities of potassium-rich foods (such as beans or leafy green vegetables); care should also be advised when used by patients who are also taking ACE inhibitors.

8 **Which of the following natural fruit juices is often recommended for the prevention and treatment of urinary tract infections?**

a) cranberry b) grapefruit c) lemon d) tomato

Although there is debate about its therapeutic efficacy, cranberry juice is often used as a potential treatment for recurrent urinary tract infections. It is believed that cranberries increase the acidity of urine, which is not suitable for the growth of pathogens and a component in cranberries is thought to prevent bacteria from adhering to the wall of the bladder. The only reported adverse effect from cranberry juice is increased diarrhoea when consumed in large volumes. Those who are not convinced about the therapeutic effect of cranberry juice suggest that the reported improvement in symptoms and prevention of infection are mainly due to the patient increasing their overall intake of fluids, which helps to flush the urinary tract regularly, thus minimizing the opportunity for infection to develop because pathogens do not get sufficient time to grow and multiply before being expelled during urination.

9 **Which of the following salt solutions may be used to relieve the symptoms of a mild urinary tract infection?**

a) sodium chloride   b) calcium chloride
c) potassium citrate   d) magnesium nitrate

A solution of alkalinizing salts – namely, potassium citrate or sodium citrate – will relieve symptoms of mild infections of the lower urinary tract such as cystitis (infection of the bladder) or urethritis (infection of the urethra). Alkalinizing solutions act by increasing the pH of the urine (making it less acidic), which relieves the discomfort caused by lower UTIs. Patients should also be encouraged to drink lots of water to flush out the urinary tract. If alkalinizing salts do not relieve symptoms, the antibiotic trimethoprim may be prescribed to treat the bacterial infection; painkillers such as paracetamol or ibuprofen may also be recommended to treat the discomfort. Most people can be treated at home for a lower UTI, but certain patients may require hospital treatment for an upper UTI, such as older people, pregnant women, cancer patients, and people who are HIV positive.

10 **The best way of monitoring the effectiveness of a diuretic is by recording:**

a) a fluid balance chart   b) weight and height

c) height   *d) weight*

From a nursing perspective, recording fluid input and output on a fluid balance chart is not always the most accurate means of monitoring the effectiveness of a diuretic, since it relies on the cooperation of the patient. The best way of monitoring the effectiveness of a diuretic is by weighing the patient regularly.

11 **Which of the following is not a form of urinary incontinence?**

a) overflow incontinence   *b) impatient incontinence*

c) stress incontinence   d) urge incontinence

Incontinence describes involuntary urination and can usually be classified as overflow, stress or urge incontinence. There is a range of treatments available depending on the type of incontinence experienced by the patient. Overflow incontinence is more common in males and is usually due to prostate enlargement. It is treatable with alpha-adrenergic blocking drugs such as tamsulosin, which relax smooth muscle; however, these drugs can cause hypotension as a side-effect. Stress incontinence is caused by weakened pelvic floor muscles and/or a weakened urethral sphincter muscle, allowing urine to leak from the bladder (see Answer 15). It is often preventable by exercising the pelvic floor muscles but where this is not sufficient, patients may be prescribed a serotonin and noradrenaline reuptake inhibitor (SRNI) such as duloxetine (more commonly used as an antidepressant). Urge incontinence is usually due to overactive detrusor muscles of the bladder walls; bladder retraining is often the first line of treatment but where this is unsuccessful antimuscarinic drugs, such as oxybutynin, may be recommended. Care must be taken when prescribing these drugs to patients with heart disease as they can exacerbate CHF.

FILL IN THE BLANKS

12 *__Loop__* **diuretics are the most potent class of diuretic.**

Loop diuretics (also known as 'high ceiling' diuretics) are the most potent diuretics, capable of inducing substantial diuresis – increasing the dose increases the level of diuresis. Examples of loop diuretics include furosemide and bumetanide. They act on the ascending loop of Henlé. They are also good venodilators (dilator of veins), which makes them useful for the treatment of acute left ventricular failure. Furosemide is the most commonly prescribed loop diuretic and increases urine output even when blood flow to the kidneys is diminished, which makes it a useful treatment for patients with renal failure. Deafness is a side-effect associated with high doses of furosemide. Loop diuretics can also induce hypotension and loss of electrolytes, namely sodium, calcium, and magnesium. Excessive loss of potassium may also be a problem with repeated use, so loop diuretics may be used in combination with a potassium-sparing diuretic (see Answer 7).

13 *Mannitol* is the diuretic of choice for treating cerebral oedema.

Mannitol is an osmotic diuretic that acts on fluid passing through the renal tubules (nephrons). It increases osmotic pressure in the nephrons of the glomerulus, which inhibits the passive reabsorption of water from the filtrate back into the blood. It is used in the treatment of cerebral oedema and is usually administered by rapid IV infusion to quickly relieve intracranial pressure due to the oedema (for example, after a head trauma). Mannitol may also be used in the treatment of raised intraocular pressure and as a remedy for drugs overdose by increasing the excretion of toxic substances. It is contra-indicated in patients with intracranial bleeding, pulmonary oedema, and renal failure.

14 The electrolyte *calcium* may be retained as a side-effect of thiazide diuretics.

Retention of calcium is a side-effect of thiazide diuretics, while loss of calcium may be a side-effect of the loop diuretics such as furosemide. Thiazide diuretics, such as bendroflumethiazide, are mainly used to treat hypertension and are less potent than loop diuretics. Thiazide diuretics act at the beginning of the distal convoluted tubule, whereas loop diuretics act at the ascending portion of the loop of Henlé. Thiazides act in two ways: by slightly increasing the volume of urine output (much less than the effects caused by loop diuretics) and dilating the blood vessels – together these effects reduce blood pressure. Side-effects associated with thiazide treatment tend to be uncommon, since the dose usually required for treatment of hypertension is quite low.

15 *Stress* incontinence is the most common type of urinary incontinence.

There are a number of different forms of incontinence but the most common is stress incontinence, which together with urge incontinence, accounts for 90% of incontinence cases. Stress incontinence is common in women who have had children, particularly if they have had several vaginal deliveries. Stress incontinence may occur in men who have had treatment for prostate cancer such as surgical removal of the prostate and radiotherapy. Other risk factors common to both genders include obesity, a family history of incontinence, and increasing age. The most common forms of treatment for incontinence are non-pharmacological and non-surgical, involving pelvic floor exercises, bladder training, and losing weight (if appropriate). When these methods are not successful, pharmacological therapies can prove effective (see Answer 11).

16 **The tricyclic antidepressant _imipramine_ may be prescribed to treat nocturnal enuresis in children who have not responded to other treatments.**

The initial treatment for nocturnal enuresis in children involves advice on fluid intake, toileting habits, diet, and behaviour. If children do not respond, then an enuresis alarm should be considered, which has a lower relapse rate than drug treatment in children who are well supported in their treatment. The TCA imipramine should only be considered following specialist assessment of children who have failed to respond to other forms of treatment (such as desmopressin alone or in combination with an alarm). Treatment should not be continued beyond three months and toxicity can be an issue. It may also induce behavioural changes and relapse is common after withdrawal of the treatment.

 MATCH THE TERMS

17 Trimethoprim   **E.** antibiotic

18 Furosemide   **C.** loop diuretic

19 Oxybutynin   **A.** antimuscarinic

20 Mannitol   **B.** osmotic diuretic

21 Desmopressin   **H.** antidiuretic

22 Potassium citrate   **F.** alkalinizing agent

23 Amiloride

I. potassium-sparing diuretic

24 Spironolactone

G. aldosterone antagonist

25 Bendroflumethiazide

D. thiazide diuretic

Figure 10.1 Drugs used to treat common disorders of the urinary system

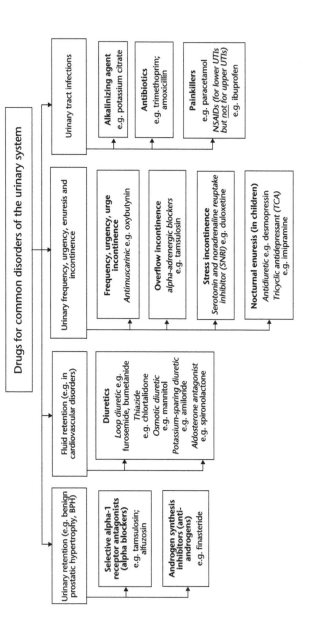

11 Pharmacological treatment of cancer

INTRODUCTION

Cancer develops due to excessive and uncontrollable cell growth. A cancerous (or neoplastic) cell develops due to a mutation in a single cell, which affects the control of normal function in the cell. The mutation allows the cell to grow and proliferate without the normal regulatory controls of cell growth and replication, and it loses the ability to enter apoptosis (cell suicide). Initially, the uncontrolled growth of the cancerous cells is localized but because such cells have lost the ability to undergo apoptosis, they do not die and so the mass of proliferating cells begins to invade nearby tissue and may eventually metastasize to other sites in the body. The majority of solid tumours arise from epithelial tissue, since epithelial tissue divides rapidly and is the main type of tissue lining the internal and external surfaces of the body's organs (for example, the lungs, colon, and breasts). Tumours arising from epithelial tissues are called carcinomas. Sarcomas originate in connective tissue, lymphomas are derived from cells of the immune or lymphatic systems, while haematological cancers are classified according to the blood cells from which they originate.

Treatment of cancers is very diverse and the options available are based on a number of factors, namely the type of cancer, location of the primary tumour, the tumour grade, presence of metastases, and the patient's general health. Nurses need to consider that there are numerous short-term and long-term side-effects from the different types of cancer treatment. They should be conscious of the high risk of infection associated with cancer treatment as well as being mindful of the patient's emotional well-being during and after treatment.

Useful resources

Nurses! Test Yourself in Pathophysiology
All chapters

Nurses! Test Yourself in Anatomy and Physiology
All chapters

Further Essentials of Pharmacology for Nurses
Chapter 3

TRUE OR FALSE?

Are the following statements true or false?

1 Many cytotoxic drugs cause vomiting a few hours after administration.

2 Mouth ulcers are a rare side-effect of cytotoxic treatment.

3 Some patients do not experience a significant therapeutic effect from antiemetic drugs used to treat chemotherapy-induced nausea and vomiting.

4 Radiotherapy is the use of high-energy radiation to kill malignant cells.

5 All of the cells damaged during radiotherapy can be replaced.

6 Trastuzumab is a hormonal treatment used to treat certain types of breast cancer.

a b
c d
MULTIPLE CHOICE

Identify one correct answer for each of the following.

7 | Radiotherapy that is administered before surgery is called:

   a) adjuvant therapy

   b) neoadjuvant therapy

   c) palliative therapy

   d) total body irradiation

8 | The pharmacological effects of antiproliferative drugs are seen in:

   a) all cells (normal and malignant)

   b) slowly dividing normal and malignant cells

   c) rapidly dividing normal and malignant cells

   d) malignant cells only

9 | Chemotherapy that is administered after surgery is called:

   a) adjuvant therapy

   b) isotopic therapy

   c) neoadjuvant therapy

   d) palliative therapy

10 | Which of the following is not a form of radiotherapy?

   a) external radiotherapy

   b) internal radiotherapy

   c) isotopic radiotherapy

   d) total body irradiation

11 The human papilloma virus vaccine is classified as what type of cancer treatment?

a) chemotherapy

b) hormonal therapy

c) individualized therapy

d) biological therapy

12 Tamoxifen is classified as a:

a) hormonal therapy that acts as a competitive antagonist

b) biological therapy that acts as a competitive antagonist

c) hormonal therapy that acts as an agonist

d) biological therapy that acts as an agonist

FILL IN THE BLANKS

Fill in the blanks in each statement using the options in the box below.
Not all of them are required, so choose carefully!

immunosuppressed	tired
cytotoxic	chemotherapeutic
total body irradiation	vesicant
hormone therapy	biological therapy
palliative	local site irradiation

13 _____ drugs carry a high risk of tissue necrosis if they extravasate.

14 Patients receiving cytotoxic chemotherapy are at increased risk of infection because they are _____.

15 Most anticancer drugs can be described as _____ agents.

16 _____ _____ _____ is a type of radiotherapy sometimes given to patients having a bone marrow or stem cell transplant.

17 _____ radiotherapy may be given to relieve symptoms such as pain.

18 _____ _____ is treatment to boost or restore the ability of the immune system to fight cancer, infections, and other diseases.

ANSWERS

 TRUE OR FALSE?

1 **Many cytotoxic drugs cause vomiting a few hours after administration**

The nausea and vomiting associated with chemotherapy are due to damage to the lining of the GI tract caused by the drugs. Cisplatin has particularly severe emetic (vomiting) side-effects, which are thought to be the result of the drug's stimulation of serotonin receptors in the GI tract and the brainstem. To overcome the emetic effects, a powerful serotonin antagonist – ondansetron – can be used as an antiemetic drug.

2 **Mouth ulcers are a rare side-effect of cytotoxic treatment**

Mouth ulcers are a very common and unpleasant side-effect of cancer chemotherapy. It is due to the effect of the drugs on the mucous membranes of the mouth, although the patient's immunosuppressed state will also contribute. A number of steps can be taken to minimize the complication: (1) before chemotherapy treatment commences, a patient should be examined by a dentist or dental hygienist to have any infections treated; (2) if the patient develops a sore mouth (or the white cell count decreases) during chemotherapy treatment, nystatin pastilles and chlorhexidine antibacterial mouthwash should be used prophylactically against *Candida* yeast and bacterial infections, respectively; (3) if mouth ulcers develop, a local analgesic spray (such as benzydamine) may be used to relieve discomfort; lidocaine gel may also be applied directly to the painful area.

3 **Some patients do not experience a significant therapeutic effect from antiemetic drugs used to treat chemotherapy-induced nausea and vomiting**

There are many different types of antiemetic (antisickness) drugs. The type prescribed will depend on whether the sickness is caused by the cancer or its treatment, and the patient's past medical history. To effectively inhibit vomiting, the antiemetic should be given before chemotherapy and, to sustain its effect, the medication should be given regularly and not just when needed. Occasionally, some patients still feel sick after taking an antiemetic drug, in which case adding another type of antiemetic may help. Some patients experience additional side-effects due to an antiemetic drug, which can sometimes be relieved by taking a different type of antiemetic.

4 **Radiotherapy is the use of high-energy radiation to kill malignant cells**

Radiotherapy works by damaging the DNA of cells in the area being treated. This causes the cells to stop growing or die. Radiotherapy is usually in the form of X-rays that specifically target the treatment site, which means normal and malignant cells in that region will be affected by the radiation. Although normal cells are also affected, they are better at repairing themselves than malignant cells, so they recover quite quickly. A course of radiotherapy is usually given over a number of days or weeks. Each treatment is known as a 'fraction'. Fractions are usually given once a day over a 5-day period (Monday to Friday) with a rest over the weekend to allow normal cells time to recover.

5 | All of the cells damaged during radiotherapy can be replaced

The ability of cells to be replaced following radiotherapy depends on the type of cell and the dose of radiotherapy. Most of the body's healthy cells that are damaged during radiotherapy can be replaced, such as hair follicles, although certain cells cannot be replaced, such as sperm and egg cells. When cells that cannot be replaced are damaged, the side-effects can sometimes be permanent (such as infertility).

6 | Trastuzumab is a hormonal treatment used to treat certain types of breast cancer

Trastuzumab (commonly known by its trade name, Herceptin®) is a monoclonal antibody which is a biological therapy used to treat breast cancers that are classified as 'hormone receptor positive', meaning they overexpress the HER2 receptor. It is only effective when this receptor is overexpressed and therefore this treatment is not recommended to patients who express normal HER2 levels, as it will have no therapeutic effect in these patients. Depending on the cancer grade, it may be used alone or in combination with a cytotoxic agent.

MULTIPLE CHOICE

Correct answers identified in bold italics.

7 | Radiotherapy that is administered before surgery is called:

a) adjuvant therapy   ***b) neoadjuvant therapy***
c) palliative therapy   d) total body irradiation

Neoadjuvant (or preoperative) radiotherapy describes radiotherapy that is given before surgery to shrink a tumour, making it easier to remove; neoadjuvant radiotherapy can also be used to reduce the risk of a tumour spreading during surgery. This type of treatment is frequently used in some cancers, such as rectal cancer. Chemotherapy can also be given as neoadjuvant treatment prior to surgery, either alone or in combination with radiotherapy. Chemotherapy and radiotherapy given together is called chemoradiation.

8 **The pharmacological effects of antiproliferative drugs are seen in:**

a) all cells (normal and malignant)

b) slowly dividing normal and malignant cells

c) *rapidly dividing normal and malignant cells*

d) malignant cells only

The faster a cell grows and replicates, the more susceptible it will be to the pharmacological activity of an antiproliferative drug because these drugs target the cell's machinery for growth and replication. Due to their antiproliferative nature, these drugs will affect all rapidly dividing cells, both malignant and normal cells. This is the reason for some of the unpleasant and sometimes distressing side-effects associated with cancer chemotherapy, such as mouth ulcers, nausea and vomiting, hair loss, and infertility. The mouth and GI tract are lined with epithelial cells, which by their nature are rapidly dividing, making them targets for antiproliferative agents. Hair cells are rapidly dividing, which is why hair loss is a common side-effect with many chemotherapeutic agents. The sex cells (gametes) are also rapidly dividing and are therefore affected by antiproliferative agents, which can have implications for the patient's future fertility. Patients who wish to have children in the future are routinely offered the opportunity for sperm or egg harvesting prior to commencing anticancer treatment.

9 **Chemotherapy that is administered after surgery is called:**

a) *adjuvant therapy*   b)   isotopic therapy

c)   neoadjuvant therapy   d)   palliative therapy

When chemotherapy is given after surgery to remove a tumour, it is called adjuvant (or postoperative) treatment. The aim is usually to kill off any microscopic tumour cells that may have been left after the operation. It is often used in breast cancer, rectal cancer, and cancers of the head and neck area. Radiotherapy may be given as adjuvant treatment, either alone or in combination with chemotherapy.

10 **Which of the following is not a form of radiotherapy?**

a)   external radiotherapy   b)   internal radiotherapy

c)   *isotopic radiotherapy*   d)   total body irradiation

There is no such treatment as isotopic radiotherapy. About 40% of cancer patients will receive radiotherapy as part of their treatment. It can be given in various ways: as external radiotherapy, internal radiotherapy or a total body irradiation. There are lots of forms of external radiotherapy. In general, external radiotherapy is applied from outside the body using X-rays, 'cobalt irradiation' or particle beams (of electrons or protons). Internal radiotherapy uses radioactive metals or liquids to damage the cancer from within the body. The radiotherapy is administered by drinking a liquid containing radioactive isotopes that are taken up by cancer cells. Alternatively, a metal material containing radioactive isotopes is implanted in, or close to, the tumour; this is called brachytherapy. In some patients, the radioactivity from a metal implant can initially be detected outside the body, so they should avoid close contact with people until the radioactivity drops to safe levels. Total body irradiation is radiotherapy applied to the whole body to eradicate the bone marrow prior to transplant (see Answer 16).

11 **The human papilloma virus vaccine is classified as what type of cancer treatment?**

a) chemotherapy b) hormonal therapy
c) individualized therapy *d) biological therapy*

Cancer vaccines are a relatively new type of biological therapy. For most cancer types, they are not yet part of standard cancer treatment and are mainly available as part of clinical trials. There are two main types of cancer vaccines: vaccines to prevent cancer and vaccines to treat cancer. The human papilloma virus (HPV) vaccine is being offered to teenage girls to help reduce the risk of developing cervical cancer (caused by HPV) later in life. It acts to prevent cancer in a similar manner to vaccinations for other illnesses.

12 **Tamoxifen is classified as a:**

a) hormonal therapy that acts as a competitive antagonist
b) biological therapy that acts as a competitive antagonist
c) hormonal therapy that acts as an agonist
d) biological therapy that acts as an agonist

The aim of hormonal (endocrine) therapy is to slow or stop the growth of certain cancers using synthetic hormones or other drugs to add, block or remove the body's natural hormones. Tamoxifen is a selective oestrogen receptor modulator (SERM) that acts as a competitive antagonist for the natural oestrogen receptors expressed in a variety of human tissues. Certain types of breast cancers express a lot of oestrogen receptors and since oestrogen stimulates breast cancer cells to grow, blocking the receptors will prevent the oestrogen from binding and stimulating cancer cell growth. Tamoxifen competes with natural oestrogen in the body to bind with the oestrogen receptors and inhibit growth of malignant cells. Like trastuzumab, tamoxifen will only be pharmacologically beneficial in patients who overexpress the oestrogen receptor (such patients are classified as oestrogen receptor positive). The main side-effects of tamoxifen are similar to the symptoms of the menopause, although it also carries a slight increased risk of secondary malignancies in the future, thus treatment is not recommended for longer than five years. Tamoxifen also interacts with warfarin.

FILL IN THE BLANKS

13 *Vesicant* **drugs carry a high risk of tissue necrosis if they extravasate.**

Sometimes injected drugs may leak out of the vein and cause necrotic damage to the surrounding healthy tissue. Vesicant drugs such as doxorubicin, epirubicin, and vincristine cause severe necrosis if they extravasate. If extravasation occurs, a full extravasation procedure must be followed — policies may vary between health care providers. Drugs such as bleomycin, are described as irritant because they can cause pain on extravasation but do not cause tissue damage. In this situation, 1% lidocaine can be administered to relieve pain.

14 **Patients receiving cytotoxic chemotherapy are at increased risk of infection because they are** *immunosuppressed***.**

Anticancer drugs depress the bone marrow, which suppresses the immune system, leaving patients at risk of developing infections — particularly minor infections that do not normally cause illness in healthy individuals. Immunosuppressed patients often respond poorly to antibacterial drugs. They must take extra care to protect themselves from infection, such as observing strict hygiene protocols, washing food thoroughly before eating, and limiting contact with potential infection (such as not visiting other patients in hospital). Nurses (and other carers) should also observe these practices when caring for immunosuppressed patients.

15 **Most anticancer drugs can be described as** *cytotoxic* **agents.**

Cytotoxic describes drugs that damage or kill cells but do not affect the underlying pathophysiology of the diseased cells. Most cytotoxic cancer therapies are antiproliferative, meaning they act mainly on dividing cells to halt their growth. Such drugs do not inhibit metastases and have no effect on tumour angiogenesis (vessel formation).

16 *Total body irradiation* **is a type of radiotherapy sometimes given to patients having a bone marrow or stem cell transplant.**

Total body irradiation (TBI) is radiotherapy to the whole body. It is very effective in killing malignant cells anywhere in the body but it also destroys the immune system and bone marrow cells. These will be replaced by bone marrow from a donor or the patient's previously harvested cells. Other normal cells will also be affected by TBI but, unlike the cancerous cells, they are able to recover. There are short- and long-term side-effects of TBI, which include nausea and vomiting, diarrhoea, dry mouth, skin rash, and swelling of the parotid glands in the neck. Most patients who undergo TBI will become infertile due to the dose of radiation. A secondary malignancy may develop in the future, although this is a rare side-effect.

17 *Palliative* **radiotherapy may be given to relieve symptoms such as pain.**

Palliative radiotherapy is aimed at controlling symptoms and providing the patient with a better quality of life. It is not aimed at treating or curing the cancer. Palliative radiotherapy is often given in fewer fractions than curative radiotherapy (or even as a single treatment), so the overall dose is lower, which reduces the side-effects yet still relieves pain. Palliative chemotherapy is another alternative to relieve symptoms; as with palliative radiotherapy, the dose of chemotherapy is not tailored to treat or cure the cancer but aims to improve quality of life.

18 *Biological therapy* **is treatment to boost or restore the ability of the immune system to fight cancer, infections, and other diseases.**

Biological therapy (immunotherapy or biotherapy) describes treatment to boost or restore the ability of the immune system to fight cancer, infections, and other diseases. It can also be used to reduce certain side-effects of some cancer treatments. Agents used in biological therapy include monoclonal antibodies, growth factors, cancer growth blockers such as tyrosine kinase inhibitors (TKIs) or proteasome inhibitors (PIs), and vaccines. Drugs that block the growth of cancer blood vessels (anti-angiogenics) are also a form of biological therapy. Biological therapy is a rapidly developing field in the pharmacological treatment of cancer.

Figure 11.1 Pharmacological and radiotherapy treatments for cancer

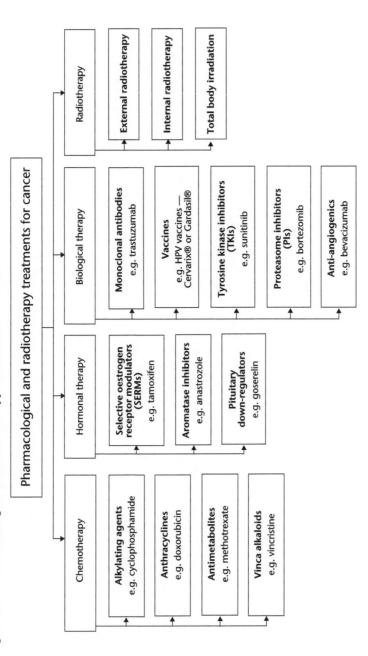

12 Drug treatment in children, older adults, and pregnancy

INTRODUCTION

When administering drugs for a therapeutic effect, it is essential that an appropriate amount of drug enters the bloodstream through which it is distributed to the desired site of action. The two main factors that influence drug concentration in the blood are the rate of drug administration and the rate of drug elimination from the body. The length of time blood takes to reach the tissues where drug action is desired depends on the amount of water and fat in the specific tissue. When administering drugs to children and older adults, it is essential to consider how the biochemistry of their organs and systems differs from that of adults and consideration must also be given to the appropriate routes of administration. During pregnancy, the increased volume of fluid in the body has a diluting effect on the dose of drug administered, although this may be counteracted by a decrease in protein binding, which leaves more free, unbound drug available in the blood. Liver enzymes also increase, which can affect the metabolism of certain drugs, while excretion by the kidneys may be increased.

Differences in age, body size, disease states, and physiology result in differences in the way the body handles the drug (pharmacokinetics), the effects of the drug (pharmacodynamics), and side-effects in children and older adults. The age-related changes in absorption, distribution, metabolism, and elimination of drugs further affect where and how much of each drug is deposited in the body and ultimately lead to alterations in dosing in both populations but particularly in children.

When administering medicines to children, it is advisable to consult the BNF for Children (published annually in July) where available, although the BNF makes certain recommendations for prescribing to children. Nurses should be mindful of the different physiological states in children, older adults, and during pregnancy, and how this can influence the choice, dose, administration, and excretion of drugs.

Useful resources

Nurses! Test Yourself in Essential Calculation Skills
Chapter 16

Nurses! Test Yourself in Non-Medical Prescribing
Chapter 8

Trounce's Clinical Pharmacology for Nurses, 18th edition
Chapter 31

TRUE OR FALSE?

Are the following statements true or false?

1 Older adults tend to have lower levels of plasma proteins.

2 A baby's liver is fully matured at birth.

3 Delayed gastric emptying in children under the age of 12 years means orally administered drugs remain in the stomach for longer.

4 The dose of drugs administered to children should never be higher than a recommended adult dose for the same drug.

5 Most drugs do not cross the placenta.

MULTIPLE CHOICE

Identify one correct answer for each of the following.

6 Which of the following does not affect sensitivity of older adults to drugs?

a) fewer drug binding sites

b) changes to hepatic enzymes

c) mobility

d) reduced organ function

7 Which aspect of the infant's anatomy allows for greater distribution of drugs into the central nervous system?

a) blood–brain barrier

b) the relatively large size of an infant's head

c) immature liver

d) lack of mobility

8 Which drug is not recommended for children under one year as it carries a risk of producing 'Grey Baby Syndrome'?

a) amoxicillin

b) chloramphenicol

c) co-amoxiclav

d) erythromycin

9 Drug interactions are more likely in older adults since they often take a number of different medications. Using multiple medicines is known as:

a) drug addition

b) drug overdose

c) drug dependency

d) polypharmacy

10 During which stage of pregnancy is the embryo/foetus at greatest risk of drug toxicity leading to congenital abnormalities?

a) implantation (days 5–15 post-fertilization)

b) embryo stage (days 15–55 post-fertilization)

c) foetal stage (day 55 to birth)

d) during labour and delivery

FILL IN THE BLANKS

Fill in the blanks in each statement using the options in the box below.
Not all of them are required, so choose carefully!

injected	high
intravenous	nomogram
transdermal	respiratory system
low	nervous system
subcutaneous	intramuscular

11 Children have thinner skin meaning they absorb _____ drugs more quickly.

12 Absorption of _____ drugs is erratic in newborns.

13 A _____ can be used to calculate drug doses for children.

14 As the body ages, the _____ _____ becomes more sensitive to certain drugs.

15 Most drugs consumed by a nursing mother are detectable in breast milk at _____ concentrations.

ANSWERS

TRUE OR FALSE?

1 | **Older adults tend to have lower levels of plasma proteins**

Older adults tend to have lower levels of plasma proteins such as albumin. This means that plasma proteins become saturated with drugs more quickly, leaving higher quantities of drug molecules remaining free and unbound in the plasma, thus increasing the plasma concentration of the drug. The increased concentration of free, unbound drug in the plasma means the patient will experience an increased drug effect. It is therefore important to monitor the older patient's compliance with medication and their response to drug treatment and nurses have an important role in educating older patients (and their carers) about such issues. Newborns also tend to have lower levels of plasma proteins immediately after birth (especially premature babies).

2 | **A baby's liver is fully matured at birth**

The baby's liver is not fully matured at birth but matures quickly in a full-term baby – usually by the age of 4 weeks. Nevertheless, care should be taken when giving drugs to babies under 6 months. Their kidneys are also immature at birth, which has an impact on renal excretion of drugs. Excretion is delayed, meaning drugs remain in the circulation for longer, during which time their pharmacological action can be augmented.

3 | **Delayed gastric emptying in children under the age of 12 years means orally administered drugs remain in the stomach for longer**

Gastric emptying is particularly irregular, unpredictable, and prolonged in newborns. The extended time the drug spends in the stomach will delay the absorption of the drug from the small intestine. A longer GI transit time means drugs also remain in contact with absorption sites for longer, meaning more of the drug may be absorbed thus leading to an increased exposure to the drug, which can enhance the drug's effect.

4 | **The dose of drugs administered to children should never be higher than a recommended adult dose for the same drug**

Total body water and extracellular fluid volume decreases with age as a percentage of total body weight. Certain water-soluble drugs, such as gentamicin, require a larger dose on a mg/kg body weight basis, when administered to neonates compared with older children or adults. This is to overcome the high volume of water in the body of a neonate, which will have a diluting effect on the drug concentration. Extracellular fluid is highest at birth but falls due to post-natal diuresis in the first 48 hours of life. Due to the differences in hepatic metabolism and renal excretion in the first few months of life, when doses are calculated according to weight, such drugs will be prescribed at relatively higher weight-related doses for children than doses recommended for adults.

5 | **Most drugs do not cross the placenta**

Most drugs cross the placenta and therefore can act directly on the developing foetus. Drugs can also indirectly affect the foetus when they interfere with an aspect of physiology in the mother's body. Drugs that cause abnormalities in the developing foetus (or are suspected of being dangerous in pregnancy) are termed teratogens. It is important that nurses establish whether a patient may be pregnant while taking their history and before administering drugs.

MULTIPLE CHOICE

Correct answers identified in bold italics.

6 | **Which of the following does not affect sensitivity of older adults to drugs?**

a) fewer drug binding sites
b) changes to hepatic enzymes
c) mobility
d) reduced organ function

As the human body ages, it undergoes many physical changes that will affect pharmacokinetics and have an impact on its sensitivity to drugs. The effects include: less effective absorption of drugs, a reduction in the number of drug binding sites, changes to liver enzymes that affect the liver's ability to metabolize drugs, less efficient distribution of drugs (because of fewer plasma proteins), and changes to the function and activity of certain organs and organ systems combined with less effective excretion through the kidneys. Together, these changes may lead to enhanced drug action, which can lead to more side-effects.

7 | **Which aspect of the infant's anatomy allows for greater distribution of drugs into the central nervous system?**

a) blood–brain barrier
b) the relatively large size of an infant's head
c) immature liver
d) lack of mobility

The blood–brain barrier is immature in infants, which allows material to pass from blood into the brain that would not enter the brain of an adult. The absence of a fully functioning blood–brain barrier allows for greater distribution of drugs into the central nervous system of the infant.

8 | **Which drug is not recommended for children under one year as it carries a risk of producing 'Grey Baby Syndrome'?**

a) amoxicillin   ***b) chloramphenicol***

c) co-amoxiclav   d) erythromycin

High doses of the antibacterial chloramphenicol are not usually prescribed for newborns and neonates due to the risk of toxicity, which can lead to Grey Baby Syndrome. This is a potentially fatal condition that can develop in neonates, particularly premature infants, due to a reaction to chloramphenicol. Symptoms include cyanosis (appearance of an ashen grey colour), listlessness, limpness/weakness, and hypotension. The toxicity is caused by a deficiency in certain liver enzymes that prevents detoxification of chloramphenicol leading to an accumulation of toxic chloramphenicol metabolites. In addition, the kidneys are not fully matured in a full-term newborn, so renal excretion of the toxic by-products of chloramphenicol is insufficient, collectively leading to an accumulation of toxic metabolites.

9 | **Drug interactions are more likely in older adults since they often take a number of different medications. Using multiple medicines is known as:**

a) drug addition

b) drug overdose

c) drug dependency

d) polypharmacy

Polypharmacy describes the use of multiple drugs to treat one or more health problems and includes prescribed and over-the-counter medicines. The risk of drug interactions increases with each additional drug taken: taking two drugs carries a 6% greater risk of drug interaction, taking five drugs carries a 50% greater risk of drug interaction, and taking eight drugs (or more) carries a 100% risk of drug interaction. Although the concept of polypharmacy applies to all age groups, it is most common in older adults who are more likely to be prescribed a number of medicines. Drugs can also interact with foods, so caution must be exercised by patients on some medications; for example, statins are contra-indicated with grapefruit, and cranberry juice is not recommended for patients on warfarin. Many medicines interact with alcohol, so it is never advisable to drink alcohol with medications at any age. Nevertheless, older people are more likely to be taking prescription drugs that interact with alcohol. They also have a reduction in their body water-to-fat ratio, which means less water to dilute the alcohol in the blood. Blood flow to the liver is reduced and liver enzymes are less able to cope with alcohol. Alcohol has a stronger and faster depressant effect on the brains of older adults, causing memory loss and problems with coordination, which can be responsible for falls and confusion.

10 **During which stage of pregnancy is the embryo/foetus at greatest risk of drug toxicity leading to congenital abnormalities?**

a) implantation (days 5–15 post-fertilization)

b) *embryo stage (days 15–55 post-fertilization)*

c) foetal stage (day 55 to birth)

d) during labour and delivery

Teratogenic damage can occur at any stage during pregnancy, although the most susceptible period is during the embryonic phase (approximately days 15–55 post-fertilization). Drug toxicity during the implantation phase usually results in spontaneous miscarriage – often before the pregnancy has even been confirmed. During the embryonic phase, the embryo undergoes most of its physical development, changing from a cluster of cells implanted into the uterus to a fully recognizable human. Due to this rapid phase of development, the embryo is particularly sensitive to drugs and toxicity may lead to congenital abnormalities. (An example is the drug thalidomide, which was used as an antiemetic to treat morning sickness in the late 1950s to early 1960s but caused severe physical abnormalities in some babies born to mothers who were treated with the drug.) During the foetal stage, the foetus continues to grow and develop, although since all of the major organ systems have developed and are now maturing, drug toxicity is less likely to cause abnormalities – although care should still be exercised when prescribing drugs during this phase. Drugs administered during labour and delivery may interfere with the baby's breathing immediately after birth and some newborn babies exhibit symptoms of drug exposure, such as drowsiness, in the days following birth. This usually wears off but in cases of respiratory depression (perhaps following opiate administration for pain relief during labour), a newborn baby may need some medical help to establish breathing immediately following birth.

FILL IN THE BLANKS

11 **Children have thinner skin meaning they absorb _transdermal_ drugs more quickly.**

Absorption through the skin is related to the thickness of the skin. Since the newborn infant has skin that is much thinner than that of an adult, drugs may be absorbed more quickly than in adults, which may lead to toxicity.

12 **Absorption of _intramuscular_ drugs is erratic in newborns.**

Intramuscular (IM) administration of drugs should be avoided in newborns and children because it may damage immature tissues. It is also very painful. Since newborns do not possess a lot of muscle or fat tissue and blood supply is increased to developing muscles, absorption of drugs administered into the muscles is quite erratic and unpredictable.

13 A *nomogram* can be used to calculate drug doses for children.

A nomogram uses a person's height and weight to calculate the body surface area (BSA), which provides a more accurate representation of an individual's metabolic processes than using body weight alone. Using a ruler, a line is drawn between the patient's body weight and height. Where the line crosses a central scale is the patient's BSA, which can then be used to calculate an accurate drug dose for a child. Alternatively, accurate paediatric doses may be recommended in the BNF for Children or a dose can be determined using the recommended dose for their weight or age (probably the least accurate, given the extreme variation in size of children).

14 As the body ages, the *nervous system* becomes more sensitive to certain drugs.

The brain and nervous system become more sensitive to certain medicines as the body ages. This makes older adults particularly susceptible to the side-effects of opioid painkillers, such as morphine and sleeping tablets such as diazepam, which act on the brain and nervous system. To reduce such side-effects, a lower dose may be prescribed for a shorter duration. Forgetfulness is also associated with advancing age, meaning older adults may have trouble with adherence and compliance, such as remembering to take drugs or remembering why certain medicines were prescribed. To help with these issues, a number of strategies can be used such as medicine reminder charts and pill boxes that can be filled with all the daily or weekly tablets required. Failing eyesight can cause problems with reading small print labels and information leaflets supplied with medicines. If this is impacting on compliance, the pharmacist should be able to supply drugs with large print labels.

15 Most drugs consumed by a nursing mother are detectable in breast milk at *low* concentrations.

Although most drugs are detectable at very low concentrations in breast milk, it is advised that nursing mothers avoid consuming any medication, as some drugs, even in low concentrations, can still be toxic to the baby or cause a hypersensitivity reaction. This also applies to the consumption of alcohol. Premature babies and those who developed jaundice are particularly at risk of drug toxicity. If it is unavoidable for the mother to take a medication, she should be advised to feed the baby prior to taking the drug because this is when the concentration of the drug will be lowest in her body. Certain drugs are contra-indicated while breast-feeding and in situations where the mother should take such medication, the safest advice is to bottle-feed the baby to protect it from exposure to the drug. A general rule of thumb when advising nursing mothers is: if it is not advisable during pregnancy, it should also be avoided while breast-feeding.

13 Drug interactions, poisoning and its treatment

INTRODUCTION

In an ideal world, drugs would specifically treat the condition they are designed for and not cause any other effects in the body. However, since the administration of medicines involves introducing chemicals into the body, and given that the body's physiology may already be altered due to illness, it is inevitable that drugs will have additional effects that may be undesirable or in extreme cases life-threatening. This is known as a drug interaction. The more drugs a person is taking, the more likely they are to experience a drug interaction. This is known as polypharmacy and is more common in older adults, since they are more likely to be taking a range of drugs for different illnesses (see Chapter 12). Many drugs exhibit a range of interactions when taken in combination with other drugs, but some non-prescription medications and even certain foods or liquids can also cause drug interactions, some of which are quite serious. Nurses have a responsibility to educate patients on the dangers of such interactions with other medications but also potential interactions that exist with everyday foods and drinks.

When a patient ingests too much of a prescription drug or accidently consumes a toxic product, they may exhibit symptoms of poisoning. Often it is not possible to identify the exact poison or the dose ingested, although this is not usually important since few poisons have specific antidotes. Where there is any doubt surrounding any aspect of a suspected poisoning, the National Poisons Information Service should be consulted.

Nurses should be familiar with common side-effects, drug interactions and be able to recognize adverse drug reactions. If a side-effect or adverse drug reaction is suspected, the Medicines and Healthcare products Regulatory Agency (MHRA) should be notified via the *Yellow Card Scheme*.

Useful resources

Nurses! Test Yourself in Non-medical Prescribing
Chapter 11

Medicines and Healthcare products Regulatory Agency
http://www.mhra.gov.uk/index.htm#page=DynamicListMedicines

National Poisons Information Service

http://www.npis.org/

TRUE OR FALSE?

Are the following statements true or false?

1 Adverse drug reactions are considered different from side-effects.

2 Most poisons that impair consciousness will have no effect on respiration.

3 Drinking too much alcohol in a short space of time can lead to poisoning.

4 The most effective treatment for suspected alcohol poisoning is to allow the person to 'sleep it off'.

MULTIPLE CHOICE

Identify one correct answer for each of the following.

5 Which of the following criteria is not used to assess the severity of poisoning?

a) circulation

b) level of consciousness

c) temperature

d) respiration

6 Stimulants, such as cocaine, can kill in three ways. Which of the following is not a mechanism by which stimulants may be fatal?

a) hypothermia

b) heart attack

c) overheating

d) brain damage

7 The usual oral dose of activated charcoal when treating an adult is:

a) 10 g

b) 50 g

c) 100 g

d) 500 g

8 When is it acceptable to alter a medication (for example, by crushing it) to help with administration?

a) if the patient consents

b) when the patient asks you to

c) if the patient does not understand why the medication is being given

d) it is never acceptable to alter the packaged form of a medication

FILL IN THE BLANKS

Fill in the blanks in each statement using the options in the box below.
Not all of them are required, so choose carefully!

---

activated charcoal	naloxone
acetylcysteine	cytochrome P450
cytochrome P250	antiemetic drugs

---

9 The amino acid derivative, _____, may be used to treat para-cetamol poisoning.

10 The antidote for treating opiate overdose is _____.

11 Oral administration of _____ _____ is an effective method of eliminating many poisons from the digestive system.

12 When the liver detects a potential toxin in the blood, it responds by altering the production of the _____ _____ enzyme specific for the metabolism of that toxin.

ANSWERS

TRUE OR FALSE?

1   **Adverse drug reactions are considered different from side-effects**

Side-effects are not considered adverse drug reactions. An adverse drug reaction describes a reaction that is always undesirable for the patient. Not all side-effects are undesirable or unwanted but can be beneficial. For example, sildenafil – more commonly known as Viagra® – was originally developed for treating pulmonary hypertension but had a positive side-effect of maintaining the male erection, a discovery that transformed its use and it is now primarily prescribed for erectile dysfunction. There are a number of different classes of adverse drug reactions but the two most common are *augmented adverse drug reactions* and *bizarre adverse drug reactions.* Side-effects experienced while taking medication are usually considered to be tolerable by patients, and include mild nausea or vomiting. However, when a side-effect is not tolerable to a patient, it may be considered an augmented adverse drug reaction.

2   **Most poisons that impair consciousness will have no effect on respiration**

Most poisons that affect consciousness will depress respiration by reducing the sensitivity of the respiratory centre in the medulla oblongata to carbon dioxide, thus suppressing the normal breathing reflex. This can cause respiratory arrest by preventing adequate oxygen from reaching the lungs. In such situations, assisted ventilation may be required (such as mouth-to-mouth or using a bag-mask-valve device). Cyanosis is a good indicator of insufficient ventilation of the lungs. Oxygen is not a substitute for adequate ventilation, although it may be administered at the highest concentration when a patient exhibits symptoms of carbon monoxide poisoning or exposure to irritant gases.

3   **Drinking too much alcohol in a short space of time can lead to poisoning**

Every time alcohol is consumed, the liver filters out the poisons in the alcohol from the blood. Alcohol is absorbed into the body much quicker than food but the body can still only process and detoxify approximately one unit of alcohol per hour, thus consuming a lot of alcohol in a short space of time limits the body's ability to process it. This means that the blood alcohol concentration (BAC) rises and the higher the BAC, the more effect alcohol will have on the body's normal physiology. At very high levels, alcohol affects the function of the autonomic nervous system that controls vital functions such as breathing, heartbeat, and the gag reflex. Therefore, excessive consumption of alcohol can depress breathing and cause unconsciousness.

4 **The most effective treatment for suspected alcohol poisoning is to allow the person to 'sleep it off'**

Even after someone stops drinking, their BAC may continue to rise, thus it is never advisable to leave a person with suspected alcohol poisoning to 'sleep it off', as their symptoms may get worse. Signs and symptoms of alcohol poisoning include confusion, vomiting, seizures, slow breathing (less than eight breaths per minute), and hypothermia. If alcohol poisoning is suspected, immediate medical help should be sought, as severe cases can result in unconsciousness, coma, and even death. Once admitted to hospital, the patient is monitored until the alcohol has left their body; they may be given IV fluids to prevent dehydration and replace lost electrolytes and in severe cases the stomach may need to be evacuated.

MULTIPLE CHOICE

Correct answers identified in bold italics.

5 **Which of the following criteria is not used to assess the severity of poisoning?**

a) circulation

b) level of consciousness

c) *temperature*

d) respiration

When a patient is admitted with suspected poisoning, it is essential to first assess if the situation is life-threatening due to airway obstruction or respiratory arrest. Once this has been determined and the appropriate action taken to stabilize respiration (if necessary), the next step in treating poisoning is to assess the severity of poisoning by determining circulation, level of consciousness, and respiration rate. Circulation is assessed by regularly monitoring blood pressure, with a low blood pressure indicating a failing circulation. Perfusion of vital organs (such as brain and kidneys) is essential, so the nurse must ensure that the blood pressure reading is not due to intense constriction of vessels, which is indicated by cold, blue peripheral regions, namely the hands and feet. Level of consciousness is assessed as one of four categories: Grade 1 – drowsy, but responsive to light stimulation; Grade 2 – unconscious but responsive to light stimulation; Grade 3 – unconscious but responds to severe stimulation; Grade 4 – unconscious with no response to stimulation. Respiration rate should be recorded on the patient's chart at regular intervals and the patient observed for signs of cyanosis, which would indicate under-ventilation of the lungs. Blood gases and the respiratory minute rate should also be measured.

6 | **Stimulants, such as cocaine, can kill in three ways. Which of the following is not a mechanism by which stimulants may be fatal?**

a) *hypothermia*   b)   heart attack

c)   overheating   d)   brain damage

Stimulants such as cocaine, amphetamines, and MDMA (ecstasy) trigger the release of the hormone noradrenaline and increase levels of the neurotransmitter dopamine. Collectively, this causes increased motor activity, increased heart rate, increased blood pressure, and vasoconstriction. These physiological changes interfere with normal homeostasis in the body and can be fatal in three ways: (1) the increased motor activity increases oxygen demand by the heart, while the vasoconstriction can lead to a heart attack; (2) altering dopamine levels can affect the body's homeostatic thermoregulatory mechanisms, and if combined with increased motor activity can lead to a dangerous increase in body temperature, potentially resulting in organ failure and death; and (3) an increase in blood pressure increases the risk of rupturing a blood vessel in the brain, while vasoconstriction reduces blood circulation in the brain.

7 | **The usual oral dose of activated charcoal when treating an adult is:**

a) 10 g   *b)* *50 g*   c) 100 g   d) 500 g

Activated charcoal is usually administered via a nasogastric tube with an initial dose of 50 g for adults and children over 12 years of age. This dose should be repeated every 4 hours. In children under 12, the dose should be reduced to 1 g/kg (up to a maximum of 50 g) every 4 hours. Administration of activated charcoal is usually more effective at reducing absorption of poisons through the GI tract than gastric lavage.

8 | **When is it acceptable to alter a medication (for example, by crushing it) to help with administration?**

a)   if the patient consents

b)   when the patient asks you to

c)   if the patient does not understand why the medication is being given

d)   *it is never acceptable to alter the packaged form of a medication*

Drugs are only licensed for use in the form in which they are packaged, thus it is never acceptable to alter a drug from its packaged form, for example, by crushing or separating a tablet. Altering the form of a drug can interfere with its delivery and therefore absorption and distribution in the body, which can have implications for its therapeutic effectiveness. If a patient has difficulty taking their medication in a particular form, the nurse should consult the pharmacist who may be able to suggest an alternative formulation of the medicine (for example, a liquid preparation rather than a tablet) and then have the prescription changed by the doctor (or other qualified prescriber). For enteral feeding, it may be necessary to crush or separate tablets if they are not available in liquid formulations. In such exceptional situations, the doctor should always be aware that the drug is being administered via this route and then document on the prescription that the drug is to be administered enterally – this makes the administration legal.

FILL IN THE BLANKS

9   **The amino acid derivative, _acetylcysteine_, may be used to treat paracetamol poisoning.**

Acetylcysteine may be used as an antidote for paracetamol overdose. When excessive quantities of paracetamol are ingested, the liver is unable to detoxify the metabolites produced as the high dose of paracetamol is broken down. The toxic metabolites can react with liver enzymes, which may damage hepatocytes. Acetylcysteine protects the liver against the effects of paracetamol overdose by binding to the toxic metabolites, protecting hepatocytes, and preventing potentially fatal liver damage from paracetamol overdose. It should be noted that the amount of paracetamol that can trigger overdose is quite low – as low as 7.5 g (equivalent to fifteen 500 mg tablets) in adults – which makes it easy to accidentally overdose on paracetamol, particularly as it can be ingested in a variety of formulations such as tablets and cold remedies.

10   **The antidote for treating opiate overdose is _naloxone_.**

Although overdose of the stronger opiates such as heroin and morphine is commonly known, it should be remembered that overdose can also occur with milder opiates, such as codeine, when large doses have been ingested. The symptoms of opiate overdose include unconsciousness, respiratory depression, low pulse rate, hypothermia, and pinpoint pupils. Naloxone is used to reverse respiratory depression and is usually administered intravenously. It has a short duration of action and therefore repeated doses may be required. In cases of respiratory arrest, full resuscitation will be necessary along with assisted ventilation. Naloxone is also the antidote used to treat neonates born with respiratory and CNS depression due to the administration of opiates (such as pethidine, fentanyl or diamorphine) to the mother during labour.

11   **Oral administration of _activated charcoal_ is an effective method of eliminating many poisons from the digestive system.**

The sooner it is administered, the more effective activated charcoal will be at reducing absorption of toxins by the GI tract. It may still be effective up to one hour after ingestion of the poison and longer for modified-release or antimuscarinic drugs. Repeated doses of activated charcoal can enhance the elimination of certain drugs from the GI tract even after they have been absorbed. It is very useful in eliminating toxins that are poisonous in small amounts such as antidepressants. If activated charcoal induces vomiting, this should be treated with an antiemetic, since vomiting will reduce the effectiveness of the antidote treatment.

12 **When the liver detects a potential toxin in the blood, it responds by altering the production of the *cytochrome P450* enzyme specific for the metabolism of that toxin.**

Certain drugs cause an increase in the activity of cytochrome P450 enzymes, which may result in a second drug being metabolized more quickly than desired, thus decreasing the bioavailability of the second drug and reducing its overall therapeutic effect. Conversely, certain drugs may decrease the activity of cytochrome P450 enzymes. This in turn may decrease the metabolism of a second drug, since there is a reduced level of its specific cytochrome P450 enzyme, which increases the bioavailability of the second drug and enhances the therapeutic effect of the second drug. Sometimes the increase or decrease in bioavailability of drugs caused by drug interactions can be dangerous. A number of common prescription and non-prescription drugs, along with some common foods, can induce drug interactions through this inhibition or increase the activity of cytochrome P450 enzymes. See Figure 13.1 for some common examples and the drugs affected by their interactions.

Figure 13.1 Mechanisms of common drug–drug and drug–food interactions

	Drugs/foods/liquids that affect activity of cytochrome P450 enzymes	Circulating levels of the drug affected by changes in enzyme activity	
Enzyme activity is INCREASED	Carbamazepine (antiepileptic)	Warfarin (anticoagulant)	**Circulating levels of drug are REDUCED**
	Ethanol (alcohol)		
	Phenytoin (antiepileptic)	Combined oral contraceptives	
		Corticosteroids (anti-inflammatory)	
	Rifampicin (antibacterial)		
	St. John's Wort (non-prescription herbal remedy)	Warfarin (anticoagulant)	
Enzyme activity is INHIBITED	Corticosteroids (anti-inflammatory)	Amitriptyline (antidepressant)	**Circulating levels of drug are INCREASED**
	Ciprofloxacin (antibacterial)	Theophylline (bronchodilator)	
	Cimetidine (H_2 receptor antagonist)	Warfarin (anticoagulant)	
		Pethidine (opiate analgesic)	
	Grapefruit juice	Statins (anticholesterol)	

Glossary

Afterload: systemic vascular resistance against which the left ventricle must eject blood during contraction. The resistance is produced by the volume of blood already in the vascular system and the constriction of vessel walls.

Analgesia: to reduce or eliminate pain.

Analgesic: medication that reduces or eliminates pain.

Antagonist: drug that blocks the action of an agonist or natural ligand.

Anti-arrhythmic: drug used to treat irregular heartbeat (bradycardic or tachycardic).

Antibacterial: a substance that inhibits the growth of, or kills, a bacterium.

Antibiotic: a substance that inhibits the growth of, or kills, a bacterium. Sometimes used to describe substances that inhibit all microorganisms.

Antibody: (immunoglobulin) protein produced by a white blood cell that binds to a specific antigen (usually a pathogen such as bacterial, viral or fungal antigen).

Anticholinergic: see *antimuscarinic*.

Anticholinesterase: drug that blocks the enzyme acetylcholinesterase which breaks down the neurotransmitter acetylcholine.

Anticoagulant: agent or drug that slows down or prevents blood clotting.

Anticonvulsant: drug that reduces the severity of or prevents seizures.

Antidepressant: drug that relieves symptoms of depression.

Antiemetic: prevents or alleviates nausea and/or vomiting.

Antifungal: substance that inhibits the growth of, or kills, a fungus.

Antigen: a molecule (usually a polysaccharide or protein) that interacts with an antibody. The term *antigen* is often used to describe a non-self, 'foreign', material, although certain antigens are generated within the body, such as the A and B antigens found on the surface of red blood cells.

Antihistamine: inhibits the actions of histamine.

Anti-inflammatory: reducing or blocking inflammation.

Antimicrobial: a substance that inhibits the growth of, or kills, a microorganism.

Antimuscarinic: drug that blocks muscarinic receptors.

Antipsychotic: (neuroleptic) drug used to treat psychosis.

Antipyretic: drug used to lower body temperature or reduce fever.

Antitussive: cough suppressing.

Antiviral: a substance that inhibits the replication of, or destroys, a virus.

Ascites: accumulation of excess fluid in the peritoneal cavity of the abdomen.

Bactericidal: antibacterial agent that kills bacteria.

Bacteriostatic: antibacterial agent that suppresses the growth of bacteria.

Broad-spectrum antibacterial: an antibacterial agent effective against a wide range of bacteria.

Contra-indicated: not recommended for clinical use.

Emetic: causing vomiting.

Enuresis: inability to control urination.

Extravasate: to exude from or pass out of a vessel into the surrounding tissue.

Gluconeogenesis: synthesis of glucose from non-carbohydrate sources such as amino acids (protein) and fats. It usually occurs in the liver.

Gram-negative: a major class of bacteria that possess a thin cell wall and an outer membrane on their surface. This class of bacteria will not retain the violet stain in a Gram's stain test.

Gram-positive: a major class of bacteria that possess a thin cell wall but no outer membrane on their surface. This class of bacteria will retain the violet stain in a Gram's stain test.

Half-life: the time taken for the blood plasma concentration of the drug to reduce by half.

Inotrope: alters the force or strength of contraction of heart muscle tissue (see *positive inotropes* and *negative inotropes*).

Negative inotropes: decrease cardiac output and slow heart rate by reducing contraction of the heart muscle. Beta-blockers and calcium channel inhibitors act as negative inotropes.

Nocturia: passing urine at night.

Nocturnal enuresis: (bedwetting) inability to control urination at night.

Polypharmacy: meaning 'many drugs'. It is used when a patient is prescribed several different drugs. It is particularly common in older adults who may be taking medications for a variety of conditions. Care must be taken to minimize/avoid drug interactions and side-effects.

Positive inotropes: increase cardiac output by stimulating powerful contraction of the heart muscle. The cardiac glycoside, digoxin, is a positive inotrope.

Preload: cardiac filling pressure (venous return to right side of the heart).

Prophylactic: to defend against or prevent disease.

Rhinorrhoea: discharge of mucus from nasal mucous membranes.

Vasodilation: dilation of blood vessels.

Venodilation: a form of vasodilation but referring specifically to dilation of veins.